HOLISTIC APPROACH TO LIVER DISEASES

Hepatitis—A Growing Epidemic of the New Millennium

Drug-Free Natural Remedies, Healing Teas, Tonics, and Supplements. Formulas From the World of Alternative Therapies and Integrative Medicine.

Dr. Jean J. Grandoit

authorHOUSE®

AuthorHouse™
1663 Liberty Drive, Suite 200
Bloomington, IN 47403
www.authorhouse.com
Phone: 1-800-839-8640

Disclaimer: This information is based upon research and the author's personal experiences. No part of this book may be reproduced without permission in writing from the author.

First published by AuthorHouse 10/25/2007

ISBN: 978-1-4343-3526-5 (sc)

Printed in the United States of America
Bloomington, Indiana

This book is printed on acid-free paper.

Contents

Healthcare in the United States is changing. The best way to help yourself and your family is to be informed about your medical needs and choices. In this premier edition, I share the information on liver diseases I have collected over the years. I hope you will use this book as your home adviser about the health of your liver, but it is not meant to be a medical book.

Today, more than one out of every seven Americans—some 30 million people—suffer from high liver enzyme. Liver disease has become an epidemic in the United States. The incidence of liver disease, especially hepatitis C, has been rising over the past several years. In my office, I see increasing numbers of patients who seek the help of different therapies to improve, cure, or prevent liver disease from recurring.

This clinician's guide will help you become medically empowered and give you the tools necessary to practice self-care. The information contained herein is based on my research and personal experience over the past 20 years in the field of natural medicine. Natural healing is not necessarily intended to replace medical care. Rather, it will inspire and motivate you to practice self-care safely. It will help you understand the importance of relationships between liver diseases, nutrition, diet, and health. Knowledge is power. Understanding natural healing, and how it interacts with allopathic medicine, is very important. Do not stop taking medications without discussing it with your physician.

As a holistic healthcare practitioner, I believe that nutrition is an important field that has frequently been neglected. Recently, there has been an explosion of interest in nutrition and hot it relates to the diseases that affect the Western world. In the 1860s when Louis Pasteur promoted the concept of microorganisms, viruses, and bacteria as the cause of disease, everyone argued with his concept—with the exception of Claude Bernard, who insisted that the milieu interior was the most important factor in disease. He argued that weakening of the immune system made humans susceptible to the ravages of microorganisms, toxins, and allergic substances. In his dying words, Pasteur—the man whose research enabled the existence of today's modern vaccines—said, "The germ is nothing; the inner terrain is everything. Claude Bernard was right; the immune system does play a role in the prevention and treatment of disease. Every month some new product is introduced that is designed to help us build a stronger immune system—the first line of defense in fighting most deadly diseases.

Natural medicine's principles have served the vast majority of the world's population successfully as long as it has been in existence. Conventional medicine, however, has been considerably less successful in treating chronic degenerative conditions, such as heart disease, cancer, and stroke (the nation's three leading causes of death), as well as other conditions that are stress related, such as asthma and chronic stomach distress.

Certainly, people on both sides of the stethoscope will benefit from the medical empowerment of natural medicine. Whether we like it or not, the future of medicine will be a combination of conventional and natural medical practices—integrated, or integrative, medicine. The good news is that since 1996, the Health Sciences Institute has conducted extensive independent research on natural remedies. The National Cancer Institute also confirms research on natural remedies to finding a cure for cancer. In addition, million-dollar drug companies have spent money on natural remedies research.

The *New England Journal of Medicine* reported several years ago that 61 million Americans sought alternative medical therapies in 1990 and visits to alternative medicine came to 425 million, compared to 388 million visits to conventional physicians. Studies further show that American consumers are using natural methods in conjunction with conventional medicine. This has prompted many conventional physicians to integrate alternative care into their practices. The future of surviving many diseases, such as cancer, looks more promising than ever. The National Cancer Institute has identified 3,000 plants that contain properties that fight cancer cells. Seventy percent of these plants are found in the Amazon rain forest.

Over 4 million American families have been touched by Alzheimer's disease, and nearly 50 percent of those over 85 will develop symptoms of the disease. Scientists in several studies in Auckland, New Zealand, and Belgium found that patients with the disease achieved significant improvements in cognitive symptoms and daily living activities, disturbances, and psychiatric symptoms with galantamine. Those with Parkinson's disease and multiple sclerosis may also benefit from galantamine. Herbal tea extract banana plants—found in the Philippines and Southeast Asia—lower blood sugar in patients with diabetes and helps them lose weight without a change in diet or exercise.

The list of health benefits from natural therapies goes on and on. To control disease is to establish functional reserves. This process, which can help our bodies better fight diseases and slow down aging, can take many years. Natural therapies have been around since day one; we need to start using them.

Human life is undergoing many change.

Such change affects our health:

Believe that life is worth living,

And your belief will help create the fact.

—William James

Men are disturbed, not by the things that happen,

but by their opinion of the things that happen.

—Epictetus

We can control our thoughts...

and by controlling our thoughts...

by using this greatest power...

the power to choose...

we are indirectly able to control conditions.

—J. Martin Kole

A strong proponent of a holistic approach to health and healing, Dr. Jean Grandoit brings to the natural medicine field his experience as a health advocate, lecturer, researcher, writer, clinician, administrator, educator, speaker, author, and consultant. He has 20 years of nutritional counseling experience in natural health, alternative, complementary and integrated medicine. He is a holistic healthcare practitioner, specializing in natural nutrition products that provide patients with the highest quality of care. In addition, he has designed individual programs that enable the body to heal itself. He is the founder and president of Brooklyn Holistic Center in Brooklyn, New York. He is also the originator of the Natural Health Talk Show on radio and television, and the author of numerous articles, columns, and publications.

He received training in Oriental Chinese Medicine, Acupuncture and Acupressure, Naturopathy, Homeopathy, Reflexology, Vibrational Medicine, Massage, Fitness, Nutrition, Herbal Medicine, Colon Hydrotherapy, Holistic Health Counseling, Weight Loss / Stop Smoking Program, Complementary, Alternative / Integrated Medicine

Bachelor of Science in Biology with minor in Spanish

Master Degree Level Courses in Counseling Psychology

Medical Sciences Courses in Adult Medicine and Health Care Sciences

Medical School Studies in General Medicine

Medical Courses in Alternative / Integrated Medicine

Emergency Medical Courses

Certify Nutritional Consultant

Certify Nutrition Analyst in Bio-Equilibrium Testing

Certify Holistic Health Practitioner and Counseling

Certify Herbology and Master Herbalist

Board Certify and Registered Traditional Naturopath

Doctorate in Oriental Chinese Medicine

Doctorate in Alternative / Integrated Medicine

Doctorate in Natural Medicine

Diplomated Integrated / alternative Medicine

Family Practice, Internal Medicine and Cardiology Physician's Associate

A poem to you, Marie Alberte Raymond Grandoit:

A DREAM OVER THE CLOUD

I sat impatiently by the door every morning waiting for you

I check with the kids to make sure you were about to appear

Nothing has happened

Nothing, I repeated in my heart, disappointed I asked the

Children where is Mammy?

I asked them straight out that morning

But something must have happened, I said

The children look at me and said nothing

I am sure, sure, sure Mammy is coming

I said, Aw man, I ain't do nothing; it ain't fair

I wait, wait, and wait...finally I realize it was a

Dream Mammy (my wife) deceased four years ago from

Terminal gallbladder cancer she will never come back to us

Again

—Jean J. Grandoit

IMPORTANT NOTE TO READERS

This manual is intended for information purposes only. It is intended to advise people to question their own health and learn for themselves. The Brooklyn Holistic Center, as well as the author, makes no medical claims—either direct or implied. The reader should consult a licensed physician for any condition that might require his or her services.

This book's mission is to help people learn and accept responsibility for their own health. It is not intended to be a substitute for any treatment or medication that may have been prescribed by your physician. Stopping the use of a prescribed medication can be very dangerous. I encourage readers to consult their physician before undertaking any form of self-care treatment.

Many nutrients in this book have not been evaluated by the Food and Drug Administration. The products mentioned here are not meant to diagnose, treat, cure, or prevent any disease. Information and statements made are for education purposes only, not intended to replace the advice of your family physician. You should not go on nutritional supplements without first consulting your family physician.

This book discusses only one aspect of liver disease: hepatitis. It shows how to live with hepatitis without any drugs, medications, and chemicals—and without any potentially dangerous side effects. This book shows that liver diseases can be prevented by alternative, complementary, and integrated therapy. It is easy to understand and easy to follow. I hope this book opens the door to understanding why we suffer from various liver disorders. I hope it shines a light on the factors that may contribute to poor health, such as lack of exercise, illegal drugs, alcohol, smoking, environmental pollutants, and most important our diet.

The Brooklyn Holistic Center does not dispense medical advice, or prescribe or diagnose illness. We design individual nutritional programs and specialize in natural nutritional products that improve people's lives. I strongly believe that every person should be armed with the knowledge of natural alternative treatment—especially when allopathic methods, including prescription drugs, have failed to deliver positive results. The promotion of health is the part of the preventive solutions people should use to take control of their own healthcare.

Many views on nutritional supplements for liver disorders are conflicting. Readers should understand that the experts may disagree. However, our grandparents may not know why some natural remedies work, but they have learned from their own experiences and have passed it on to us.

The World Health Organization estimates that two-thirds of the world's population use herbs as their primary medicine. In addition, the ancient civilizations of Africa, India, the Middle East, Greece, and Europe obtained relief from herbal medicines. Today, most of us use herbs without realizing it. Even most herb critics use herbs. And do not forget that 25 to 35 percent of all prescriptions now have plants and herbs as active ingredients, including aspirin (mistletoe), menthol (peppermint), children's cough syrups (wild cherry bark) and bensodent (allspice), just to name a few.

Today, we continue to benefit from the healing power of plants and herbs, just as people did some 60,000 years ago. As we continue to learn about them, it becomes more and more evident that interest in herbal medicine throughout the world is increasing.

In spite of the fact that the effects of many herbs have not been proving scientifically, many physicians in Europe and China use herbal medicine in their everyday practice.

Angels, Angels, Angels, Angels, Angels, Angels

I knew my heavenly father had sent them from above.

There are angels all around us. We just have to believe

that with their love and guidance, there's

nothing we can't achieve.

—Frankie Vasquez

I have a special angel, who watches over me.

He keeps me out of trouble, from, sets me free.

—Paula R. Harbacek

Only God could send them here to keep me in his care.

Now I'm content just knowing that there are

Angels everywhere.

—a passage of Nancy Watson Dodrill from the Angel Datebook 2003

THIS BOOK IS DEDICATED TO THE MEMORY OF:

Eliane Elie—My beloved mother, who passed away from a cerebral vascular accident stroke on July 27, 1998. She spent a good part of her life gathering green medicine (herbs) to treat my brothers and sisters, as well as me, and I know she is always with us.

Marie Alberte Raymond Grandoit—My wife, who passed away from gallbladder cancer on February 2, 2000. She filled my life with love and helped me keep my life together during the years of writing.

Jean Lionel Grandoit—My godchild and brother, who passed away from a heart attack in his sleep on January 4, 2001. He made natural medicine part of his life. He is always in my heart.

Jean Hiram Grandoit—My father, who passed away in his sleep on August 8, 2002. He always reminded me that herbs have many secrets and that we can learn much about their uses for prevention and cure.

To all my friends, clients, and mothers of natural medicine:

I am indebted to those who have encouraged me to develop my thinking in writing this book and who have helped bring this project to reality.

To the Lord Jesus Christ:

I am particularly grateful because I know he cares for me and is always by my side to direct my path. He has never rejected my prayer or withheld his love. I give him thanks and praise every day.

Finally, I pray for those who are in the dark. Know that you will see the light. Your eyes will be opened; just believe in the Lord Jesus Christ and he will bring you into his way. He will lead you down a straight path from darkness into the light.

For those: Let food by the medicine and they medicine food.

—Hippocrates

The doctor of the future will give no medicine, but will interest his patients in the care of the human frame, in diet, and in the cause and prevention of diseases.

—Thomas Edison

May God be with you as you strive for healthy life. Your body you know is the temple of the holy spirit who is in you since you received him from God. You have been bought and paid for. This is why you should use your body for the glory of God.

—Corinthians 6:19–20

For the earth which drinks in the rain that often comes upon it, and bears herbs useful for those by whom it is cultivated, receives blessings from God.

—Hebrews 6:7

I went down into the garden of nuts to see the fruits of the valley...

—Song of Solomon 6:11

As a child, I was very ill with chronic anemia and dizziness. My parents always brought me to see a physician who used botanical medicine in his practice. Because of this, I have long been attracted to herbal medicine. In 1975, during my first year of medical school in Louvain, Belgium, my daughter was born in Boston, Massachusetts, with the problem of chronic vomiting. She vomited all foods and liquids. In the vast majority of children, if this problem is not resolved, it can lead to abdominal surgery, disability, or death. We saw medical specialists, but her condition continued to deteriorate.

In 1978, my wife and I took her to a botanical practitioner in Brussels, Belgium. The practitioner placed her on a specific carbohydrate diet and gave her herbs and nutritional supplements; within six months, she was free of symptoms. A few years later, she began to eat normal foods and liquids; she has been in excellent health every since.

Since having that experience with my daughter, I became convinced that we can improve our health through natural remedies. There is much we can do to keep our health at optimum levels so we live long, healthy lives. As I developed more interest in botanical medicine, I became an integrated / alternative holistic medical practitioner. In 1988, I opened my private practice, Brooklyn Holistic Center, and founded Natural Health Talk TV.

The good news today is that many people are aware of their medical problems and the need to change their lifestyle. I believe knowledge is power, and everyone should learn everything they can to learn to take control of their health.

ACKNOWLEDGMENTS

Thanks to my hardworking sharp-eyed team at the Brooklyn Holistic Center Monica, Joan, Fegon, and Edna, my natural health talk show co-speaker, and little Johanseen (two years old), who carries my writing papers from one side to the other. Above all, as my friends, they have been ideal companions, critical and challenging as well as encouraging and supportive. I thank them for their long hours of work on the manuscript as well as the premier issue of natural health talk show on liver disease.

Thanks to my friend Dr. Antoine Archille, an integrated / alternative physician who has helped me, both directly and indirectly, in the writing of this book.

Thanks to many wonderful friends for keeping me company on the telephone every night for more than two and one-half years. Because of them, I was never lonely.

I thank especially my children: Albert, Janouska, Sachandra, and Janathan. I appreciate their help and support. Their continual encouragement was important to this project.

I owe thanks that cannot be expressed in words to my late wife, Marie Alberte, who inspired me with her own personal experience with natural remedies and who always encouraged and reminded me that I must follow my heart and study what is the most important in my life. I am grateful for her constant support.

I would like to acknowledge the contributions my patients have made to my writing this book. I have learned so much from them, and would like to express my affection and gratitude. Deep appreciation goes to the many physicians with whom I have worked and who have contributed their time and support, as well as their expertise on advances in therapy for chronic hepatitis C. They truly have helped further the understanding between Western and natural medicine.

Finally, this book is dedicated to people living with liver disease, especially hepatitis. I hope to provide them with what they need to know so they may come to terms with their liver disease.

Alternative medicine refers to any form of medicine that is outside the mainstream of orthodox medicine. Alternative medicine exists in all cultures. The term "natural medicine" is used to cover all forms of unrelated nonorthodox therapeutic practices. The following list includes known forms of medicine:

- Complementary medicine
- Alternative medicine
- Integrative medicine
- Traditional medicine
- Unorthodox medicine
- Holistic medicine
- Ethno medicine
- And so forth

The holistic approach involves the health and well-being of body, mind, and spirit. In contrast, orthodox medicine concentrates solely on the mechanical aspects of the body. Alternative and complementary therapies are used in place of allopathic medicine; these have not been proven by traditional scientific investigation. These therapies are not only provided by medical doctors but by other healthcare professionals with different initials after their names and different training backgrounds.

In a 1993 survey, the Center for Alternative Medicine Research at Boston's Beth Israel Deaconess Medical Center found that one in three adults in the United States use some form of alternative medicine to prevent illness. The study provided the surprising information that Americans spent $13.7 billion on unconventional therapies in 1990 and made an estimated 37 million more office visits to alternative practitioners than to primary care doctors. Seventy percent of patients never told their primary care physician about their use of alternative therapies. In 1996, the study reveals that $3.24 worth of herbal remedies were purchased.

Research shows that alternative and complementary therapies are used most often in the United States to treat many different illnesses. In Europe and elsewhere, complementary medicine serves as a supplemental therapy. Are these therapies safe? Which one helps which problem?

The fact is, both doctors and patients are in the dark. There is a death of scientific data available about the safety and efficacy of most alternative treatments. Until more research is available, alternative therapies tend to be unproven by allopathic practitioners. But people today who use nonconventional remedies when they are seriously ill will continue to use them, and most still will not discuss their use with their physician. Many physicians, in fact, are quick to dismiss their patients' interest in them.

This has not impacted the popularity of nonconventional treatments. Many explanations have been offered in regards to their popularity. One is that many doctors are in the dark about the safety or efficacy of most alternative treatments.

In 1992, the National Institutes of Health (NIH) established an office of alternative medicine. Its purpose is to evaluate alternate therapies. The office defines complementary and alternative medicine as a broad domain of healing resources that encompasses all health systems, modalities, and practices, and their accompanying theories and beliefs. CAM defines all such practices and ideas as preventing or treating illness or promoting health and well-being.

Alternative therapies include, but are not limited to, the following disciplines:

- Folk medicine
- Herbal medicine
- Diet fats
- Homeopathy
- Faith healing
- New age healing
- Chiropractic
- Acupuncture

- Naturopathy
- Massage
- Music therapy

In 2002, the Medical Subject Headings (MeSH) section staff of the National Library of Medicine classified alternative medicine under the term *complementary therapies*. This is defined as therapeutic practices that are not currently considered an integral part of the conventional allopathic medical practice. Therapies are termed as *complementary* when used in addition to conventional treatments and as *alternative* when used instead of conventional treatment. Alternative/complementary medicine are used together with orthodox medicine. Everyone can be helped with holistic alternative / complementary therapies. If you have not found hope or help with a chronic condition or illness, you should look into holistic alternative medical treatments.

In general, the digestive system includes the mouth, salivary glands, esophagus, stomach, small intestine, large intestine, liver, gallbladder, and pancreas. Each plays a specific role in digestion (figure 1).

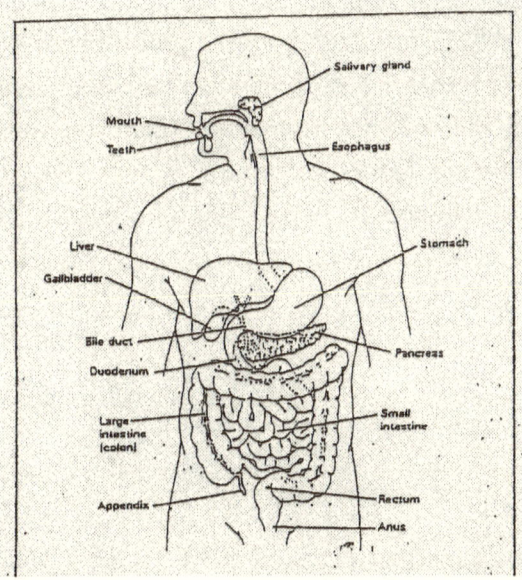

The abdomen contents extend up below the rib cage and down into the pelvis. Palpitation of the abdomen can reveal more information than the chest. It is useful for anyone interested in liver problems to know that the abdomen is divided into four quadrants made by a vertical line (the mid line) from the xiphoid process to the symphysis pubis, and by a horizontal line across the umbilicus.

The quadrants (figure 2) are as follows:

- Right upper quadrant (RUQ)
- Left upper quadrant (LUQ)
- Right lower quadrant (RLQ)
- Left lower quadrant (LLQ)

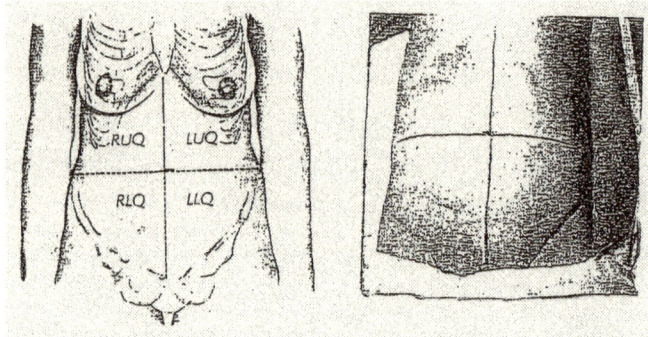

For proper examination of the abdomen, the patient should be lying comfortably in the supine position, with his or head supported by a pillow. The patient's arm should not be raised since this position tends to stretch the abdomen muscles, putting them under tension and making the abdomen harder to examine.

The examiner should develop a habit to inspect the abdomen from all angles (figure 3).

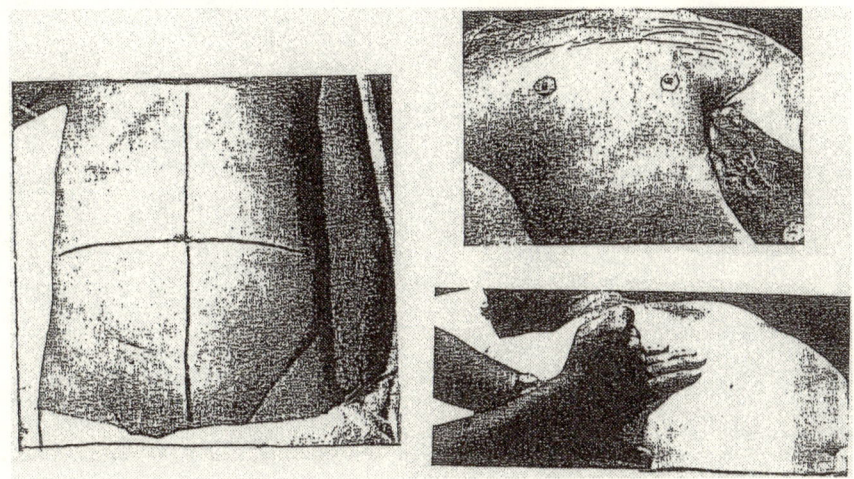

The liver as well as the spleen, kidney, and stomach all move by descent of the diaphragm on inhalation and intestines downward, producing outward motion of the upper abdominal wall. In men, this motion is much more pronounced on average than in females. The abdominal contents extend below the rib cage and down into the pelvis (figure 4).

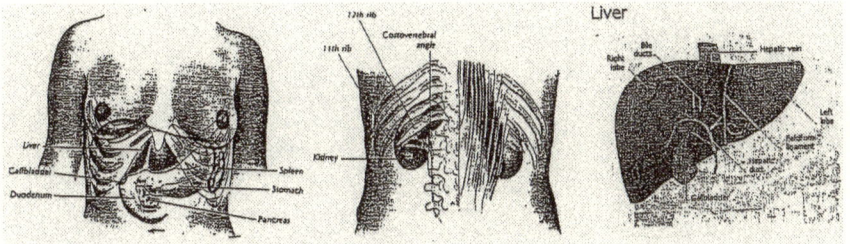

A normal liver weighs about 1200 to 1600 grams (figure 5).

Here our focus is on the liver; therefore, examination of the liver is very important. The normal liver often extends down just below the right coastal margin in the upper right side of the upper abdomen and is connected to the stomach, large and small intestines, and gallbladder. It may be palpable in the right upper quadrant, but usually on a deeper level lie the lower pole of the right kidney and the gallbladder, located on the underside of the liver. The liver and gallbladder work together with the bile ducts to help the body rid itself of waste and processed fats. This is why the liver and gallbladder are called miraculous organs. In order to feel the liver, you may have to alter your pressure according to the weakness and resistance of the abdomen wall. The liver weighs from 2 to 3 pounds and is shaped like a cone; it is reddish-brown in color.

In prehistoric times, the human race lived free from illness. Today, about 90 percent of the population in modern society die each year from disease—a result of imbalanced modern life. Poor diet and nutritional deficiencies in the Western diet that is high in fat, carbohydrates, additives, and preservatives, and low in fiber leads to improper elimination and constipation. This leads to waste accumulation and a build-up of toxins, which leads to liver disease—a serious condition that is related to the digestive process.

The gastrointestinal tract is a 25- to 32-foot tube that begins at the mouth and ends at the anus. As mentioned earlier, the digestive system includes the mouth, salivary glands, esophagus, stomach, small and large intestines, gallbladder, and pancreas. Each plays an important, specific role in digestion—especially the gallbladder, pancreas, and liver, which are part of the accessory organs.

The liver is the largest internal organ, and it is so important that it is sometimes called the master chemistry laboratory of the body. The liver has many functions that are vital to the body. Its chief function is to detoxify and remove toxic substances from the body. The liver performs many other functions as well, including processing foods and regulating vitamins and hormones (such as estrogen). When toxic or harmful substances are taken into the body, the liver converts or neutralizes it. But when the liver reaches toxic overload, that's when problems occur. Drugs, alcohol, and environmental pollutants cause congestion, which prevents the liver from eliminating toxins. The liver filters toxins from about 1 liter of blood every minute. Toxic substances attack us from all directions—in the food we eat, the air we breathe, the water we drink, as well as substances that are absorbed through the skin. A properly functioning liver can play a critical role in determining overall health.

The liver center for detoxification facilitates digestion, detoxifies poisons, produces proteins and cholesterol, stores the fat-soluble vitamins A, D, E, and K, and produces bile, which is essential for the absorption of fats. It also stimulates the small intestines, where most food absorption takes place. The liver creates bile, which aids in the digestion of fats and helps eliminate waste. It absorbs glucose or blood sugar and stores it in the form of glycogen. It assists in the breakdown and metabolizing of fats. It also helps track down red blood cells. The liver is a great reservoir of blood. It stores the blood and regulates the amount to be circulated by the heart. About one quarter of the oxygenated blood from the heart flows into the liver through the hepatic artery and other artery branches to provide oxygen to all the liver cells.

The liver works with many other organs. It works with the gallbladder to perform the functions of the biliary system. It works with the kidney to help clean the blood of poisonous substances and toxins. It is vital to helping a woman's body to process estrogen. If estrogen is not processed properly, women may have an excess of estrogen in the body, which will create premenstrual symptoms. The liver performs about 500 vital functions in the body. Most importantly, the liver can restore itself—even after half of it has been damaged.

MODERN CHINESE MEDICINE AND THE LIVER

Traditional Chinese medicine is a 4000-year system of unifying power of body, mind, and spirit. The Chinese believe in a life force, or vital energy, called *qi* (chi), which is rooted in the energy flowing through all things. The main function of the liver is to maintain flow of qi, which then circulates throughout the body as vital energy.

The most important factors about qi are the food and drink we consume and the air we breathe. This is why modern Chinese medicine regards the liver as the chief organ of the body, which allows energy to flow smoothly through the body. The liver is the detoxification center for the body. And when the liver is not functioning well, it impacts all other organs. As mentioned earlier, liver congestion is very common—especially in our polluted society where inner cleansing is overlooked.

Liver congestion or distress can manifest as a pathological disorder and lead to abdominal bloating, emotional liability, constipation, chronic candidiasis, fatigue, menstrual disorders, nausea, sore itching eyes, small red spots, skin discoloration (jaundice), and cirrhosis (scarring). Liver congestion is also caused by excessive stagnation, excessive amounts of fat sugar (converts to fat in the liver), white flour products, and chemicals found in water, food, and air. Liver overload affects the eyes, causing cataracts, night blindness, near- and far-sightedness, glaucoma, and other eye problems. Liver stagnation may cause circulatory problems and goiter. Growths, such as cancer and tumors, are caused by liver and colon congestion from lack of fiber and eating rich junk food. Most diseases, in fact, are caused by colon and liver congestion.

The Chinese also view the liver as the house of the human soul, which is said to enter the body at the moment of birth. For them, the liver is a reservoir of blood, providing blood and qi to the muscles, tendons, ligaments, nails, and eyes. It influences the ability to sleep deeply, detoxifies the blood, produces bile and enzymes, controls blood sugars, and impacts circulation and the immune system. The liver maintains both the physical and emotional balance of the body.

The Chinese even have an endearment for dear or sweetheart, *xin gan*, which literally means "heart liver."

Modern Chinese medicine differs from Western allopathic medicine. The Chinese concept recognizes that the body knows what it is doing and has its own intelligence. Therefore, a Chinese herbal doctor examines the patient's entire body; assesses the patient's complete physical and mental makeup, general lifestyle, and daily habits; and determines his or her conformation at both the physical and spiritual level. This is unlike Western medicine, wherein doctors prefer to deal with fixed concepts and absolute laws, and are focused on actions. In other words, Western doctors diagnose problems relying primarily on physical pathways and prescribe specific therapies for that problem; they do not look at the true nature of the disease.

In traditional Chinese medicine, the primary function of the liver is to maintain a flow of qi and blood throughout the body. Signs and symptoms are the basis for diagnosis, including examination of the tongue. Many people have deficiencies in their liver's function and are not aware of the problem. However, there is no single pattern within Chinese medicine that encompasses all the possible clinical presentations associated with the liver. But for those who use the integrated/alternative approaches with traditional Chinese medicine believe Chinese herbal products aim to help the body correct itself. It is an old tradition Chinese medicine concept, drawn directly from Taoist philosophy, that nature contains all the solutions to health problems. This ancient belief should always be kept in mind when using Chinese herbal medicine.

The majority of the public is still largely unaware of the chronic hepatitis that exists. It's one of the key causes of liver disease in the United States. Almost 4 million Americans, or 1.8 percent of the U.S. population, have antibody to HCV (anti-HCV). This causes an estimated 8,000 to 10,000 deaths annually. The medical establishment does not seem to have taken notice yet. Chinese medicine not only places emphasis on the liver itself, but it also places importance on hepatitis C and recognizes it as a major health problem in China. It pays to improve the health of the liver and promote detoxification.

A CHANGING MEDICINE

In this century, and particularly in the past 50 years, we have witnessed significant changes in the way medicine is practiced in this country. With that in mind, medicine, by its very nature, is preoccupied with what is wrong. Patients visit doctors when they problems; doctors attempt to identify and treat those problems. In the 21st century, we have seen fundamental changes in the demographic structure of American society. Self-care now accounts for more than 80 percent of healthcare. The real family practitioners are non-doctors as millions of people use herbs, foods, and supplements as a form of self-therapy.

Our best hope is prevention. Still, some will argue that conventional medicine uses drugs as a way of improving our health. But now we have the arrival of deadly, "smart" bugs that do not respond to antibiotics or other modern treatments. We need to place more focus on the importance of good nutrition to preserve good health and prevent disease. The human body is built from and repaired by what we eat, drink, and breathe.

In 1974, with I first became interested in alternative medicine, it was difficult to understand why the father of medicine—Hippocrates (born B.C. 460)—emphasized the role of diet in the control of disease. Yet only 70 years have passed since the first vitamins were identified. Today, we are continuing to learn about the foods, herbs, and nutritional supplements that nurture our bodies and spirits. It has become evident that alternative medicine can improve health, vigor, and vitality. Educating ourselves on how to prevent illness doesn't mean abandoning our trust in allopathic ways. Traditional medicine has its place. But there is sufficient evidence that diet and nutrition are linked to disease prevention. Therefore, individuals must take responsibility for their own health. No one knows your body better than you do.

You are your own best doctor. Take control of your health and use preventative medicine as the first line of defense in preventing disease.

Liver disease is one of the leading health problems in the world. It's the leading cause of death of people between the ages of 25 and 59 and has impacted millions of Americans. Unfortunately, many people with liver problems are not aware they have a problem until it's too late because the symptoms of liver disease often become noticeable only after a long period of time.

Every year more than 500 billion pounds of industrial waste of manmade pesticides and toxic chemicals such as formaldehyde, lead, cadmium, mercury, PCP, exortic acids, dioxin, and arsenic are produced in the United States. This is more than 1 ton of toxic chemicals for every man, woman, and child. Not only that, but most of the poisons end up in our food and water and in the air we breathe. This all poses an extreme threat to the liver.

According to one doctor in a New York State environmental study: "Everybody in the USA has detectable levels of toxic environmental pollutants, toxins, prescribed drugs, over-the-counter medications, alcohols, and chemicals produce waste accumulation which cannot filter by the liver destroy hundreds of thousand of liver cells. All those toxins overburden the liver, leading to its degeneration over time."

Although this book will primarily cover hepatitis, cirrhosis, and cancer, there are many serious illnesses that affect the liver:

- Alcohol liver
- Biliary atrasia
- Gallstones
- Gilbert's syndrome
- Hemochromatosis
- Hepatitis A
- Hepatitis B
- Hepatitis C
- Primary biliary cirrhosis
- Primary sclerosing cholangitis

- Toxic hepatitis
- Wilson disease
- Alpha one antitrypsin deficiency
- Autoimmune hepatitis
- Cirrhosis of the liver
- Fatty liver, galactosemia
- Type one glycogen disease
- Liver cancer
- Neonatal hepatitis
- Reyes syndrome
- Sarcoidosis
- Tyrosinemia
- Liver transplantation
- Liver biopsy

JAUNDICE

One of the most serious of illnesses affecting the liver besides cirrhosis and cancer is hepatitis. Hepatitis is a viral infection of the liver, which is characterized by jaundice.

WHAT IS JAUNDICE?

Jaundice is a yellowish discoloration of the skin and whites of the eyes. This condition is caused by an excess of bilirubin in the bloodstream. The liver filters bilirubin from the bloodstream and excretes it into the bile ducts, which carry it to the gallbladder. The bilirubin then flows into the small intestine.

Jaundice is not a disease but a sign of problems. Evaluation should be done with careful consideration.

Jaundice can be classified into three categories: prehepathic, hepathic, and posthepathic. Prehepathic may be caused by hemolytic anemia. Hepathic is because of the damage to the liver cells themselves from, say, hepatitis, alcoholism, and certain drugs. Posthepathic is caused by obstruction to bile transport by gallstones or cancer of the head of the pancreas.

Jaundice mostly occurs when bile is prevented from being discharged into the intestine by an obstruction. The obstruction may cause gallstones, pancreatic tumors, or parasites in the bile ducts. Jaundice may also result from drug reactions or liver diseases, including viral infections such as hepatitis, cirrhosis, and cancer that spread to the liver. Occasionally jaundice appears if too many red blood cells are too rapidly destroyed and bilirubin is released into the bloodstream as a result of a hemolytic anemia condition (prehepathic), and the liver cannot accommodate the excess. When jaundice occurs, the liver has become enlarged and is functioning less. Bowel movements may be clay colored and urine can vary in hue from light yellow to a brownish green. Skin color ranges from lemon yellow to dark olive green. If you notice any of these types of symptoms, consult your primary care physician immediately. When the liver becomes very hard, this is a bad sign and immediate attention is called for.

Treatment will determine the cause of the jaundice. Unless a backup of bile is observed, the problem could be quite serious and require surgery. Risk factors for liver disease as well as family history, certain anemia, gallbladder disease or recent gallbladder surgery, and toxic liver damage from past alcohol abuse must be taken into consideration.

Investigations of complementary medicine in the treatment of jaundice are not clearly defined. If you have jaundice, it might be best to discuss with your healthcare practitioner what the best therapeutic approach or combination of approaches might be best suited for you. But there are some general suggestions that have proven successful through my years of experience in private practice. Remember, although medical intervention is necessary, natural medicine can also be used during the recover phase to help prevent the recurrence of jaundice.

A juice fasting for one or two weeks, along with fresh lemon enemas, is important. (Some naturalists recommend the use of a coffee enema instead.) Drink a glass of warm water with the juice of one lemon each morning. Carrot juice, beet top and beet juice with dandelion and black radish extract are all good for rebuilding and cleansing the liver. Avoid all fried and fatty foods, eating a diet that is 75 percent raw food. Never consume raw or undercooked fish, meat, or poultry. Do not consume any alcohol.

Place castor oil or warm packs over the liver. Helpful herbs for jaundice include aloe, balsam, carrot, chamomile, dandelion, fennel, horsetail, hops, Indian yarrow root, nettle, parsley, peach leaves, red root, rose hips, St. John's wort, sonel, milk thistle, vervian, and yellow root. Take 4000 mg vitamin C twice daily with plenty of water, even during fasting. Also take brewer's yeast, as directed on the label, 50 mg vitamin B5 daily, 100 IU vitamin E daily (some practitioners order up to 1000 IU daily), and 500 mg L-glutatione/L-methione daily on an empty stomach for protection of the liver.

Hepatitis is a viral infection of the liver that was first recorded in the B.C.E. 500 to 380 time period in Talmud and Hippocrates. Since the time of the Romans, hepatitis has plagued the armies of Rome, Napolean, World War I and II, Korea, Vietnam, and Desert Storm. Today, hepatitis is emerging as the leading disease of the liver. It is estimated by the Food and Drug Administration (FDA) that hepatitis C alone kills 8000 to 10,000 Americans annually, and the death rate is expected to triple in the next two or three decades, exceeding the death rate associated with AIDs. About 1 million people in the United States are infected with HIV and one third of them are also infected with hepatitis C. According to the Centers for Disease Control and Prevention, only about 350,000 of those infected have been diagnosed.

Physicians need to test those people who are at a high risk of hepatitis. This group includes anyone who received a blood transfusion or organ transplant before 1992 because they could have been infected with the disease. Those who have injected drugs even once; shared needles to apply tattoos; shared scissors, nail files, or toothbrushes contaminated with infected blood; surgeons or other medical workers who perform invasive procedures; children born to mothers who have hepatitis C infection; people with evidence of chronic liver disease or had unsafe sex with infected partners are also considered at risk for the disease and should be tested. The virus sometimes does not exhibit noticeable symptoms for up to three decades.

HEPATITIS A

Figure 6 shows a man with yellowing skin and eyes, signs of hepatitis A.

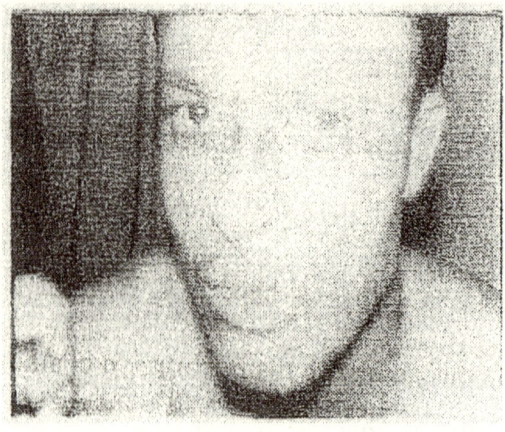

JAUNDICE

Jaundice is not a disease but a sign of several problems, including blood or liver disorders, or the consequences of a tumor, gallstone, or surgery.

Jaundice causes the skin to take on a yellowish or greenish tinge.

Figure 7.0.   Figure 7.1

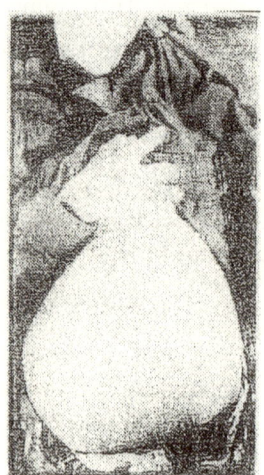

The whites of the eyes take on a yellowish color (Figure 8).

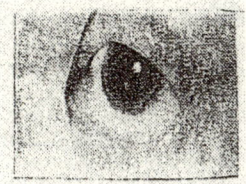

Traditional Chinese Medicine and Hepatitis

Traditional Chinese medicine encompasses all the possible clinical presentations associated with hepatitis, including:

- Examination of the tongue
- The character of the pulse
- Abdominal evaluation
- Other observations, such as retention of the damp heat, invasion of the spleen by damp, stagnation of liver chi, disharmony between the spleen and stomach, and abdominal diagnosis

No system of medicine puts greater emphasis on the liver than traditional Chinese medicine. Let's take a look at each step in more detail.

Examination of the Tongue in Hepatitis

Throughout time, the tongue has been a very important diagnostic tool in Chinese medicine. Tongue diagnosis dates back to the Shang Dynasty, which began in B.C. 1600 and ended around 1000.

This is quite different from the American view of examination of the tongue. In Chinese medicine, the examination of the tongue is done in natural light to achieve a more accurate evaluation. An acupuncturist or herbalist will, in the mind's eye, see the tongue with several different maps. Each map is shaped by the diagnostic model, or system, that it represents. The tongue should be moist and pink without any coating. It's the mirror of the body; any abnormalities can be an indication something is wrong in the body. This is why when examining the tongue, a Chinese doctor looks at the general appearance and color of the tongue; its size and shape; and the thickness of its coating or color of the tongue fur. A healthy tongue will be pink, much like a kitten or puppy's tongue, and moist, with a thin clear or white coating.

In the case of hepatitis, a sticky tongue is noted. The tongue's coating is best described as moss or fur, indicating excess because the disease has reached the lesser yang stage, or deficient yang. In some people, a red tongue with irritation and irregularities along the edge could indicate an overheated liver or sluggish overburdened liver. Most people with chronic hepatitis C tend to get high acid in the stomach, causing a fiery red tongue. This also suggests excess heat in the system.

The way a tongue appears in diagnosis does not always indicate the location of the disharmony, but the practitioner must look at other factors as well. Food, beverages, or drugs may change the coating or color of the body of the tongue. A complete evaluation of the tongue is necessary to determine the presence of acute febrile and gastrointestinal diseases.

In traditional Chinese medicine, the digestive organs are represented along the center of the tongue (figures9). *The Yellow Emperor's Classic of Internal Medicine,* Chang Chung-Ching's treatise on febrile diseases, covers tongue diagnosis in great detail. There are many other books written on tongue diagnosis.

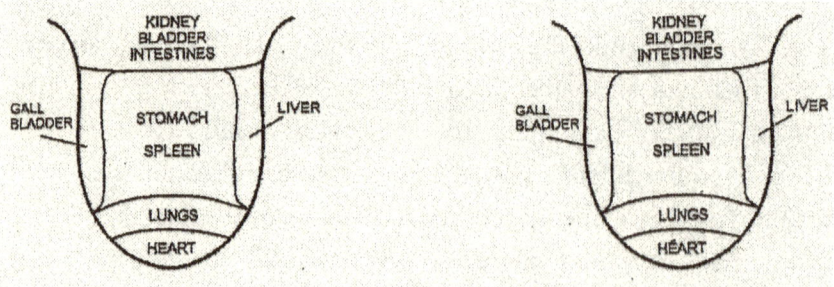

The diagram on the left represents the internal organs (figure 9). The center diagram represents the body as having three parts: upper burner, middle burner, and lower burner. The diagram on the right represents the body as having two parts: interior and exterior.

THE PULSES DIAGNOSIS IN HEPATITIS

According to traditional Chinese medicine theory, there are over 30 different pulse qualities that are essential for evaluation and diagnosis. Some Chinese medicine doctors place more emphasis on 28 pulse qualities.

Chinese pulse diagnosis is a dedicated art and difficult to master. To learn how to read pulses requires years of study and practice. Learning to interpret the pulses diagnosis means a commitment to practice the techniques on a regular basis. Feeling the pulse is a skill all of us have and one that we use every day. Since I have a degree in Oriental medicine, I practiced feeling the pulse on thousands of patients, which gave me the momentum and practice to make it a positive, effortless habit. This is why pulse evaluation must be done by a doctor trained in Chinese medicine.

Pulse diagnosis emphasizes points rather than the Western medicine focus on the frequency rhythm and density of the pulse. It's important for your healthcare practitioner to talk to you about pulse diagnosis; you should familiarize yourself with the terminology as this is key to an understanding of pulse diagnosis. It's best to perform pulse examination in the early morning, before the patient has eaten or exercised. Those activities will cause the pulse to fluctuate, rendering the physician unable to detect yin negative or yang positive. There are no absolutes to pulse diagnosis.

The examination of the pulse by Chinese practitioners is done by the doctor placing his or her first three fingers along the radical artery of the patient's wrist to feel for three special points. There are a total of six pulses on each wrist for a total of 12, which corresponds to the condition of each of the 12 organs. The normal pulse is palpable at the middle level at about four or five beats for each inhalation and exhalation of breath. They are evaluated as superficial, middle, and deep level. Of the 30 pulses known in Chinese medicine, I will emphasize the four most important:

1. Floating pulse

2. Sunken (submerged pulse)
3. Weak (slow or late pulse)
4. Bounding (fast pulse)

Floating pulse is felt under the skin with light palpation. It is an indication of an external disease—mostly yang. Sunken pulse is usually felt on heavy pressure, an indication of internal disease—mostly ying. Weak pulse beats less than 60 times per minute, as an indication of cold diseases. Patients with a weak pulse need a purgation formula to eliminate toxins in their body. Bounding or fast pulse is more than 90 beats per minute, indicating firm, hot diseases and the presence of fever in the body.

In the case of hepatitis, soft rapid pulse, soft pulse, wiry pulse with thready pulse in chronic stage of hepatitis.

The method of reading pulse diagnosis in traditional Chinese medicine is a very sensitive diagnostic technique. Even Chinese doctors, after years of practice, believe it impossible to fully master this technique. Those who do develop the expertise in reading pulse diagnosis deserve the utmost respect.

PULSES DIAGNOSIS IN HEPATITIS

Pulses are felt at the inside of the wrist where the hand and arm meet (figure 10). The first pulse is at the wrist crease on the radial side of the medial aspect of the forearm over the radial artery. The other two are proximal to the first. Together they are 28 qualities of pulse we must be on the alert for.

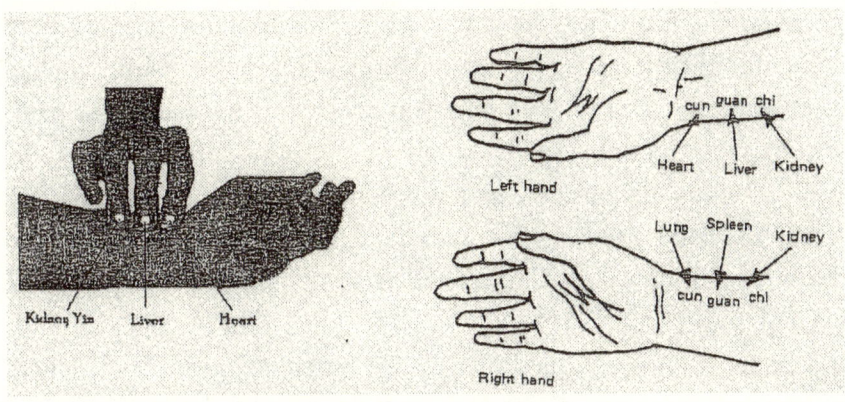

Signs and Symptoms of Hepatitis in Traditional Chinese Medicine

There is not one or a specific combination of signs or symptoms that encompass all possible clinical presentations associated with viral hepatitis. However, some etiologies or pathogeneses (*bing ji,* attributed to the evils of heat and damp. Damp heat obstructs the passage of the bile, causing jaundice; the retention of damp heat causes bright yellow skin and yellow sclera in the whites of the eyes. The accumulation of dampness obstructs movement of fluids in the body, contributing to fullness of the chest and abdomen, nausea and vomiting, deep yellow urine, bitter taste in the mouth, sticky tongue coating, and soft rapid pulse. The correct choice upon diagnosis is to clear the heat and eliminate the damp and toxins.

The effect of the repletion of the heat can impact the functioning of the spleen, causing dampness. Long-term heat along the course of the liver and gallbladder channels and interruption of the function to the spleen by dampness may cause invasion of dampness into the spleen. Consequently, the accumulation of dampness can cause a white tongue coating; slow, soft, and slippery pulses; epigastric discomfort; abdominal distention; anorexia; thirst; and scant dark urine and loose stools.

Treatment is generally to clear the damp heat and invigorate the spleen, which has been damaged. When the system is imbalanced, stagnation of the liver chi is common. This leads to symptoms of uncomfortable feelings, low-grade fever, wiry pulse, white tongue coating, bitter taste in the mouth, pain under the ribs, sharp chest pain, abdominal distention, and dry stools.

Abdominal diagnosis, which was first practiced in Japan, was not given the same attention by traditional Chinese medicine as pulse diagnosis. But now both Chinese and Western medicine use abdominal diagnosis.

There are several questions to ask when a patient experiences abdominal discomfort; many observations can be made when performing abdominal diagnosis. In both types of medicines, it requires years of practice for a physician to master the art of abdomen examination. It's a learning experience, just as it is in pulse diagnosis. After 18 years in the field of alternative medicine, I am still learning much about the abdomen. (For more details on the abdomen, refer to the appendix.)

Many centuries ago, according to traditional Chinese medicine theory, the relation between the vital organs was the key factor in diagnosis of the causes and treatments of diseases. These vital organs are the five solid and the six hollow organs, as well as the three points— or triple warmer—consisting of the openings to the stomach, small intestine, and bladder, along with the pericardium, the sack surrounding the heart. These organs are divided into five pairs. First, we have the five solid, or ying, organs: heart, lung, liver, kidney, and spleen. Then we have the five hollow, or yang, organs: small intestine, large intestine, gallbladder, bladder, and stomach. Every part of our body is affected by these vital organs and dominated by the five elements principle, which I will not discuss here. (Please see the appendix for a list of books on this topic.)

In Western medicine, evaluation of the abdomen is done by sequence: inspection, palpation, percussion, and auscultation. However, palpation of the abdomen produces more information about the location of pain because of the soft tissue structures. Pain and its location are the most important elements in the examination of the abdomen. This informs the doctor the kinds of actions that need to be taken, depending on the source of the pain. It may be serious—or it could be nothing. It is essential to determine whether the pain is somatic, involving the external parts, or visceral, involving the internal organs.

The patient will likely be asked several questions. Where is the pain? What is it like—sharp or dull, steady or colicky? When and how did it start? Is it acute or severe? (This can indicate whether it is a perforation or rupture.) How long does it last? (If it is intermittent, it could indicate acid-pepsin disease and gallbladder problems; if it persistent, it could mean peritonitis or tumor.) What makes the pain better or worse? (If the pain it better when eating, it could indicate a peptic ulcer; if the pain worsens when eating, it could mean pancreatitis or small bowel obstruction.) On respiration and movement, is the pain worse? (This may indicate problems with the liver, gallbladder, spleen, or peritonitis.) Does the pain radiate to other parts of the body? (Knowing the radiation pattern is very important for localization of pain—e.g., gallbladder [RUQ], right upper quadrant or epigastric pain area on top of the shoulder; ruptured spleen [LUQ],

left upper quadrant to top of the left shoulder; upper GU areas [esophagus, duodenum, gallbladder, biliary tree, pancreas], lower anterior chest pain possibly caused by angina, pancreatitis, gastric or peptic ulcer. Pain in the epigastric area to the middle or upper back may be an indication of perforation. In the perumbilical region, which then shifts after several hours to the right lower quadrant, rules out appendicitis. If there is pain throughout the upper chest to the back, down the abdomen and into the legs, one can rule out dissecting thoracic aortic aneurysm and dissecting abdominal aortic aneurysm. Problems with the kidney could manifest itself in flank pain, and ureters, renal colic, stone. Taking into account past medical history as well as any current medications or treatments is also important.

In the case of liver diseases, there is a specific formula. The disease progresses through various stages. And it's important for a good practitioner to find all the signs and symptoms with all the deficient that the patient is presenting and treatment must be done according of the best approach of formulas that will worked to slow down the progression of the disease.

The liver is the most crucial organ in the body, with myriad internal metabolic actions. The liver performs the following functions:

- Controls and balances blood sugar levels
- Controls the excretion and the production of cholesterol
- Maintains hormonal balance
- Metabolizes carbohydrates, proteins, and alcohols
- Regulates fat stores
- Manufactures bile and blood-clotting agents
- Stores vitamins and minerals

The liver also acts as a filter, to keep blood free from toxins, and neutralizes poisons. This one of the reason, traditional Chinese medicine refers to the liver the center for detoxification. For them, the liver regulates the body so that chi flows smoothly throughout all the meridians and all the organs. And when the liver becomes affected as a result of a disease, the whole body and energy become affected and out of balance. In hepatitis, for example, the liver functions have been compromised, the ability of the body to produce adequate immune response against those foreign invaders and hepatocellular regeneration is compromised.

For traditional Chinese medicine the liver could be the most important organ in the body. It is necessary to view many of his cause merely as symptoms of the diseases needs to clear and eliminate the damp heat evil toxins and poisons in the body. In doing so, the liver can be protected against dangerous toxins, many of its functional parts will be well balanced, and it will produces immune factors to boost the immune system. The liver is the only organ in the body that can regenerate itself when damaged. Using the preventive/integrated medicine is still the best approach dealing with individual of liver diseases.

As I write this, there is a new study that examines traditional Chinese medicine, but each interpretation is different. I highly recommend researching the topic. Please refer to the Chinese texts listed in the appendix. Deep appreciation goes to the Center for Chinese Therapy and the International Institute of Chinese Medicine, both of which have helped further my understanding of Chinese medicine.

Acupuncture in the Treatment of Liver Diseases

I have studied and practiced Chinese herbal medicine, including acupuncture, since 1986, and have seen tremendous change. More and more people, including those in the medical profession, have interest in this form of medicine. Over the years, I have intensively studied Chinese herbal therapy, which I became more interested in and have used every day in my practice. Many people come to my office with chronic pain, and I have referred them to doctors using acupuncture. The results have been good.

Now we see the enormous amounts of publicity for acupuncture in the media. Licenses in the United States were practically impossible to obtain in the 1980. Now they are many schools of acupuncture accredited and licensed in the United States. The cause of this transformation is simple: Acupuncture makes no sense but it works and has helped many people with a variety of different illness. It is remarkable today to see how the practice of acupuncture has become increasingly popular over the past twenty years. One can argue that the failure of modern medicine and the dissatisfaction of the public have generated the enormous interest in acupuncture. I disagree. I believe the interest initially began because acupuncture relieves pain and addiction control without dangerous side effects.

What Is Acupuncture?

Acupuncture is a medical therapy used for the prevention of disease. It involves the nsertion of disposable needles of varying lengths into specific points on the surface of the skin, to stimulate or disperse the flow of energy within the body. Sometimes acupuncturist apply heat (hermal heat), moxibustion, the placement of a smoldering Plug of the herb mugwort on a meridian point and by pressing, by massage, cupping in which heated cups are placed on the skin. This process produces a suction force to boost circulation and improve health.

When and where acupuncture started is not known. However, the legendary Nei Ching indicates the earliest book on the subject dates to the time of the Yellow Emperor Huang Ti (Warring period, 475 to 221 B.C.) Others were written in the time of Huang Ti (Yellow Emperor, 2674 B.C.). Early copies of this book first appeared in the Han dynasty (A.D. 206). Another book that records primitive stone instruments for acupuncture is The Book of Mountains and Seas, the Shan Hai Fing, written more than 2,000 years ago. Methods for treating diseases began in the Chou dynasty (1128 B.C.). Today, one of the most important factors is the development of acupuncture in the Western world as more and more conventional physicians refer patients to well-trained and experienced acupuncturists.

In the case of liver diseases, acupuncture provides symptomatic relieve to reduce or abolish the intra-abdominal pain that may come from the liver and others organs pancreas, gall bladder or heart. It's essential for the acupuncture practitioner to think of the underlying diagnosis, not to treat only the symptoms. This may delay the patient in obtaining effective treatment for his or her illness. In my experience, if you have located and relieved the right itself, and the pain disappears automatically. By treating the right meridians, this is regarded as second nature. And it's necessary for the patient to believe acupuncture is not a panacea or cureall. It is a therapy to stimulate or awaken natural power within the body. It's believed that energy circulates throughout the body along pathways called meridians.

The meridians are channels of thin membranous wall, filled with a transparent, colorless fluid and encircled by blood. Each of the main meridians has branches that supply with energy that supply others areas while others reach the skin's surface. Each meridian has a point of entry and a point of exit. Energy, which is a constant dynamic force circulates throughout the body, enters the meridian at the point of entry, and flows through the point of exit, where the cycle repeat again for the succeeding meridian and so on.

The Stomach Meridian descending flow of energy is being running from the head to the foot of a series of 45 bilateral points.

The Liver Meridian ascending flow of energy is being running from the foot to the chest of a series of 14 bilateral points.

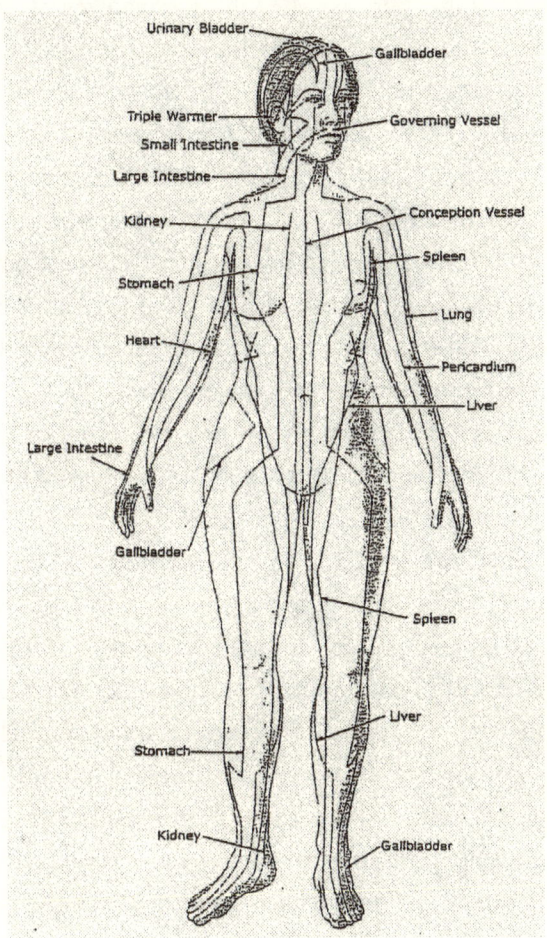

The meridian system sequence of energy flow from the lung, large intestine, stomach, spleen, pancreas, heart, small intestine, bladder, kidney, heart constrictor, triple heater, gallbladder, and liver.

Acupressure Therapy in the Treatment of Liver Diseases

Acupressure uses finger pressure on the acupuncture points to manipulate energy imbalances. The Chinese believe that the use of the hands tends to promote a feeling of mental serenity, for the blood flowing to the hands lessens the pressure on the brain and the vital energy, known as qi (chi), is the main source who keep our body functioning, keep us alive and provides the life force of all living things.

Acupressure works by using the technique: smoothing or pushing, rubbing or pain pressing, picking and finger pressing or thumb pressing on specific points that are located along the meridians. The manipulations of those points can either disperse, strengthen, or calm the vital energy qi (chi) within the body to flow.

Acupressure is very safe, with no negative emotional or physical reactions to the treatment. It can be performed whenever and wherever it is convenient. It is a very easy treatment. However, the patient may experience some light reactions to the treatment if the practitioner reached the deep root of a chronic problem. These symptoms are short-lived Understanding how acupressure works requires knowledge of the meridians and pressure points of thousands of years of practice. However, you can get started on using acupressure whenever and wherever it is convenient. The only equipment you and your partner need is a pair of hands. Wear loose, comfortable clothing to allow freedom of movement and to show better the positions of the pressure points. Self-treatment of acupressure may not possible. You need an experienced qualify acupressure practitioner who can feel the quality of qi (chi) beneath the surface of the skin.

There are many conditions under which acupressure treatment should not be given, such as in pregnant women; people with high or low blood pressure; or those with open wounds or on anyplace where there is inflammation, scars tissue, boils, blisters, rashes, or varicose veins. The young—including babies—can benefit from acupressure, but before using herbs and oils on them it's best to consult an experienced practitioner.

For liver disorders the use of acupressure and herbs with preventive measures, including diet, exercise, acupuncture, and meditation may strengthen the immune system, conquer fatigue, and help the liver against jaundice and other liver disorders.

CHINESE ACCUPRESSURE POINTS
FOR THE IMMUNE SYSTEM

St 36
This point tonifies to strengthen qi (chi) and blood circulation to protect the body from infection. It is four finger widths below the kneecap, outside the tibia.
B 13
This point is level with the third and fourth thoracic vertebrae. Tonify to strengthen the lungs.
B 20
This point tonifies to stimulate the spleen, the source of qi and blood. It is level with the eleventh and twelfth thoracic vertebrae.
B 23
This point tonifies to stimulate the kidney qi, the source of yin and yang. It is level with the second and third lumbar vertebrae.

CHINESE ACUPRESSURE POINTS FOR JAUNDICE

Cv 12
This point is below the tip of breast bone
GB 34
This is in the depression on the outside of the leg, below the knee joint, just below head of fibula. This point tonifies to calm liver qi and remove damp and heat.
St 36
This is found four finger widths below the kneecap, outside the tibia. On the lateral side in adults. St 36 is tonify to stimulate the digestive

system and relieve frontal headache by dispersing smooth the flow of qi.

Others points:

Liv 8

At the medial side of the knee posterior.

Sp 4

On the inside arch, medial side of the foot.

Gv 9

Over the eighth thoracic vertebra.

B 19

One inch bilateral to the I I" thoracic vertebra

Weak digestion, loss of appetite, indigestion, nausea, and stomach acidity with pain could be a problem in people with liver disorders. Those following acupressure points can be used:

Two Specific Points for Treatment of the Liver

GB 24

Located at the edge of ribcage on the level between tip of the sternum and umbilicus.

BIB

Two fingers widths on either side of the spine. One inch bilateral to tenth thoracic vertebra.

The ear is one of the organ not fully understood of all of the organs of the body, and this surface contains points for every single part of the entire human body. In acupuncture ear points results vary.

Ear points: Liver, sympathetic, Shen-Men, internal secretion, and gallbladder.

The method of treatment in acupuncture should be done according the severity of the disorders.

- Dispersion: requires a strong action.

- Acute: one treatment daily, and as needed.
- Chronic: One treatment every three or four hours days in total of seven treatments for one period of treatment and may be continued for three to four periods.

Many Chinese medicine practitioners called acupressure the ancient therapy. Acupuncture without needles has evolved from the same root as the Oriental arts of shiatsu and acupuncture, which we will discuss next.

WEAK DIGESTION AND LOSS OF APPETITE, INDIGESTION, AND NAUSEA

B20

This point is level with the eleventh and twelfth thoracic vertebra. When tonified, it strengthens the spleen, helping in digestion and the formation of qi and blood.

B23

This is at the level with the second and third lumbar vertebrae. It's a point that when tonified increases kidney yang, the source of body warmth, and helps digestion.

Cv12

This is located above the navel on the mid-line of the belly. When dispersing he stimulate the Spleen and Stomach, stop vomiting and move stagnation. Also helps relieve indigestion and nausea.

Liv 13

This is below the eleventh rib, at the side and bottom of the rib cage, in line with the hip bone. Disperse this point to move stagnation and to stimulate the spleen. Also helps relieve indigestion and nausea.

St 25

This is located two thumbs widths either side of the navel. Dispersing them stimulates the stomach, as well the circulation of the bowel.

Understanding acupressure is to know how to use of thumb and finger pressure on specific points to deliver the flow of vital energy for relief of the symptoms of common ailments. We will never try to do so in the way that the ancient Chinese did, nor will we use it to try to replace licensed professional healthcare. Rather, one must understand how acupressure treatment done and why it is essential to our health. It takes years to master acupressure points well, but a skilled practitioner can help to restore the harmony of body, mind, and spirit. Also, it revitalizes of the flow of energy, which is essential to our health and fundamental to the practice of acupressure.

I am not here to teach you how the channels and pressure points work or to give treatment lessons on acupressure. There are many school of acupressure in United States, all teaching different techniques for applying pressure points.

Figures 12 through 16 show some key points in acupuncture and acupressure with needles and electricity, which some use in hepatitis and jaundice.

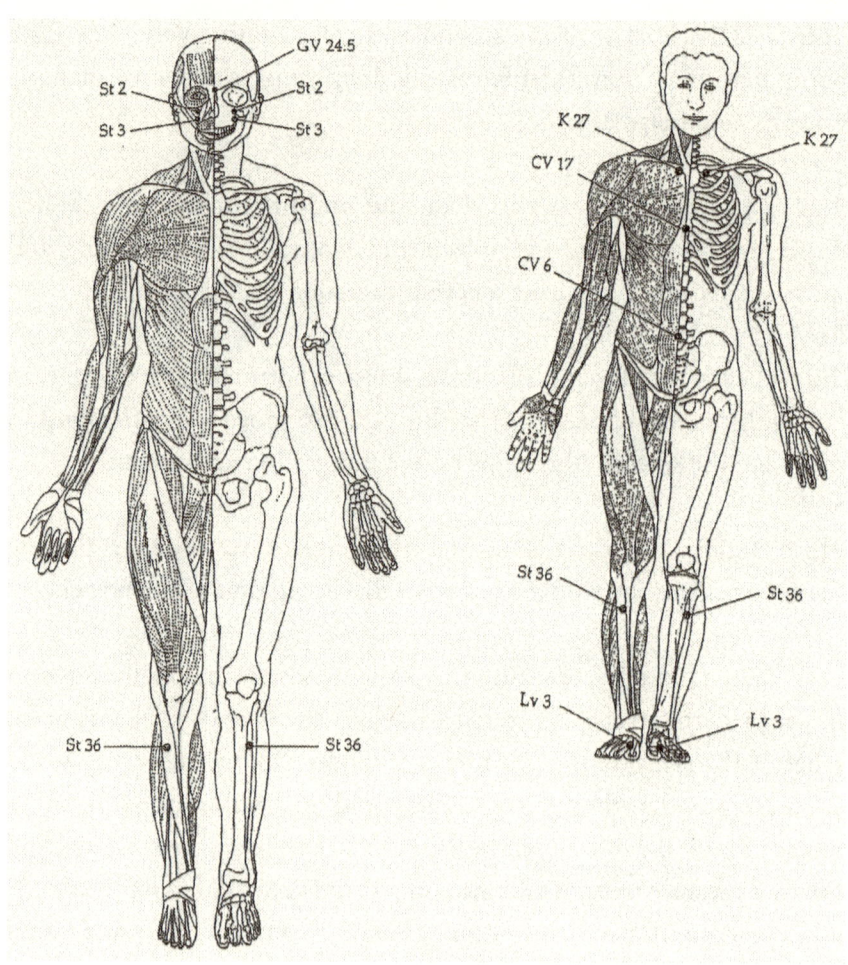

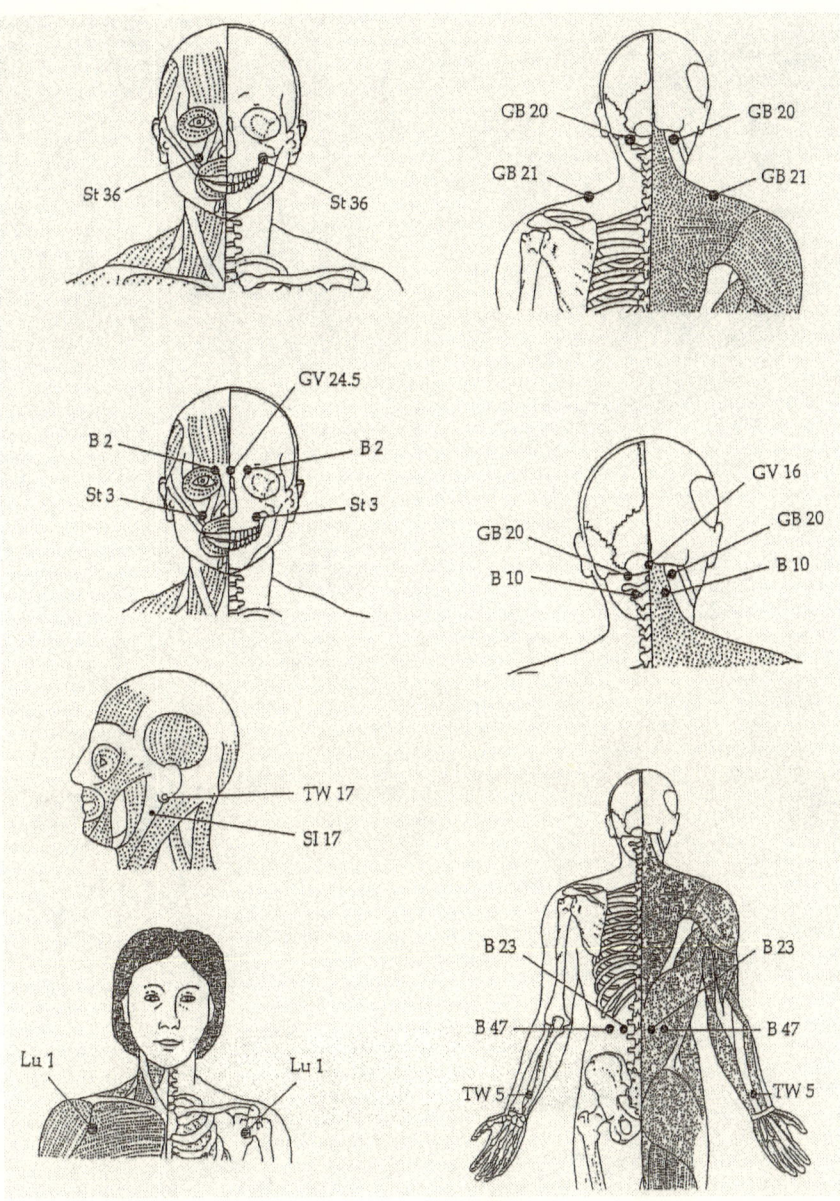

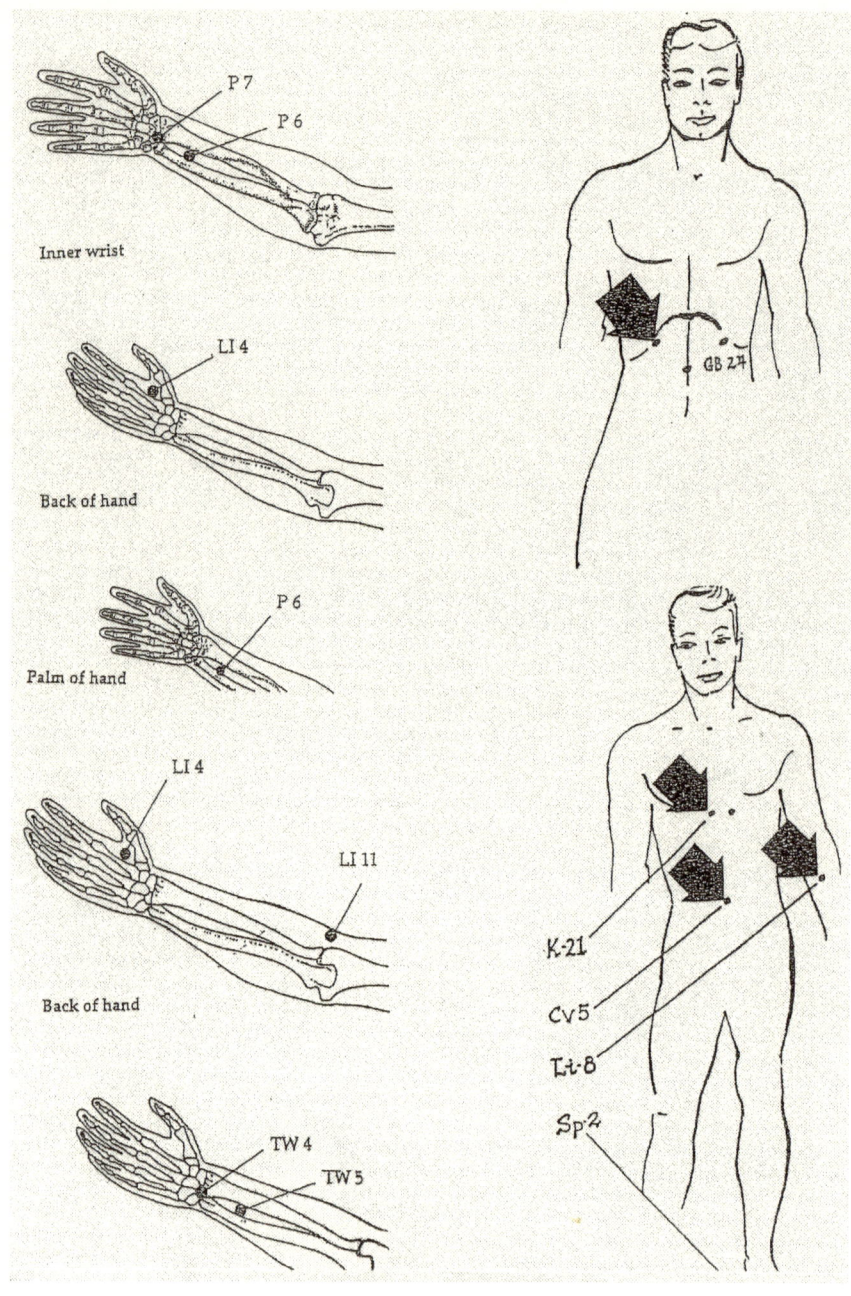

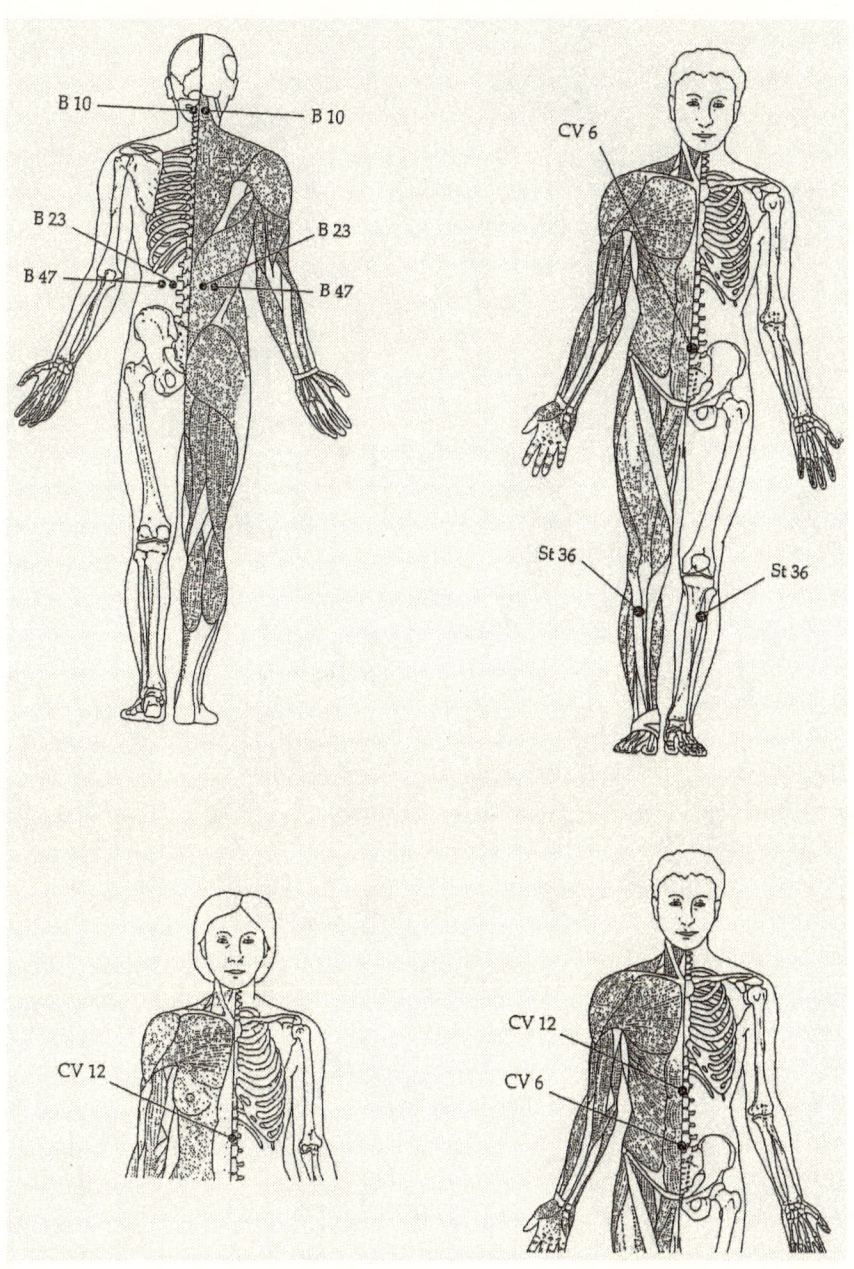

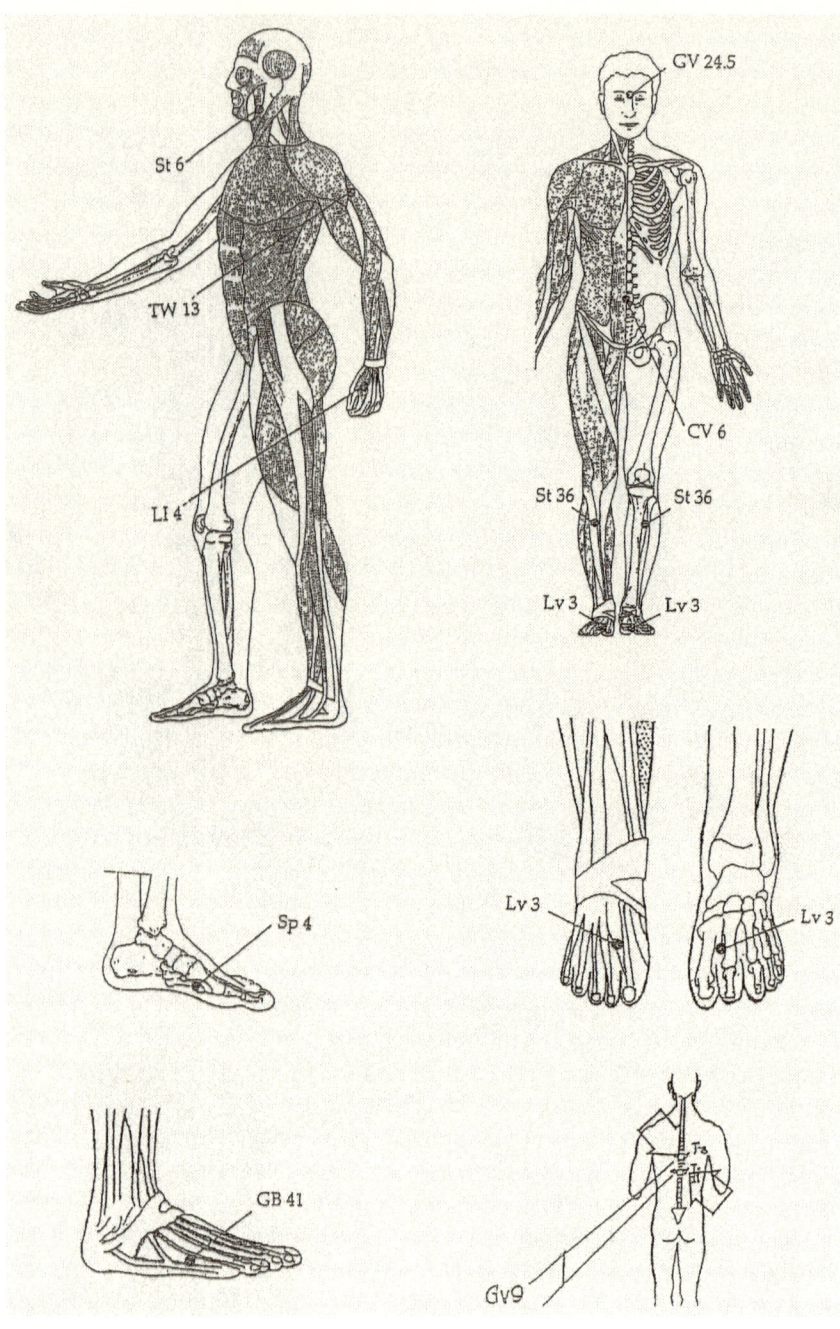

Practical Approaches in Managing Hepatitis

Overview of Hepatitis

Hepatitis comes from the Greek: *hepat* = liver; *it is* = inflammation. Inflammation of the liver is caused mostly by the hepatitis viruses or cirrhosis. It can also be caused by protein deficiencies viruses, bacteria, parasites, weak metabolism, and exposure to toxic chemicals and certain drugs.

The disease is caused by several viruses: hepatis A, B, C, D, and G. These viruses attack cells in the liver and cause diseases with many common characteristics. The way the diseases are transmitted and their outlook are substantially different, however.

Type A (infectious hepatitis) passes through the digestive tract and is spread from person by poor hygiene, contaminated food or water, or through the develops anicterus hepatitis. With the onset of jaundice, there is yellowish coloration of the skin and the whites of the eyes, dark urine, and pale stools for about two weeks. In some cases, the clinical picture can vary, from asymptomatic infection without jaundice into fulminant hepatitis, a severe condition that is often fatal.

Most people with acute hepatitis B will recovery fully. It may take up to six months and relapse may occur during that time. But if there is presence of HBsAg in the blood for more than six months, the body's immune system is unable to eliminate the virus and the person becomes a chronic carrier of hepatitis B and is very highly infectious. There are two types. First is chronic persistent hepatitis B, the more common type, which is often asymptomatic. Symptoms include fatigue, abdominal pains, weakness, fever, and intolerance to fat or alcohol. Some people never develop severe liver disease but a few may progress into the second type, chronic active hepatitis B. Their histological findings tend to be more severe. Its consequences are characterized by progression to cirrhosis of the liver and hepatocellular carcinoma (a form of liver cancer).

Type C (infectious hepatitis—HCV) is one of the most important viruses that affects the liver. The test for this virus was developed in 1989. Most experts now feel this newly discovered strain is very common in the United States. It is responsible for clinically significant cases in about 10 to 20 percent of acute hepatitis, 60 to 70 percent of chronic hepatitis, and 30 percent progression to cirrhosis (irreversible scarring of the liver), and end-stage liver disease. About 1 to 5 percent develop liver cancer. It is estimated 4 million people in the U.S. population currently are infected with hepatitis C (anti-HCV), which usually happens through contact with infected blood. It causes an estimated 8,000 to 10,000 deaths annually. And about 1,000 people each year will get liver transplant because of liver failure.

Although hepatitis C infection is spread primarily by contact with blood and blood products, most of the unexplained cases of hepatitis C transmission may happen without any known exposure to blood or to drug use. The transmission route could be from the major high risk groups for hepatitis C: People who use cocaine; injection drug users, particularly those who share needles—including those who used drugs briefly many years ago; infants born to HCV-infected mothers; people with high-risk sexual behavior, such as multiple partners; people who had blood transfusions before June 1992; and people frequently exposure to blood products, including patients with hemophilia, solid-organ transplants, chronic renal failure, or cancer patients on chemotherapy.

Another groups which hepatitis C has become a growing killer is HIV patients. It is estimated about 1 million people in the United States are infected with HIV, and a third of them are also infected with hepatitis C. The problem is that most of the people who have both HIV and hepatitis C die of AIDS before any signs of liver damage became evident. That makes diagnosing hepatitis C more complicated, hence difficult to treat. All HIV patients should be tested for hepatitis C. The best approach to confirm that diagnosis is the recently introduced test HCV RNA, which uses a sensitive polymerase chain reaction (PCR) assay. The HCV RNA is usually present and confirms the diagnosis. Others tests, such as the recombinant immunoblot assay (also called Western Blots), PCR amplification, quantification of HCV RNA in serum, genotyping and stereotyping of hcv, normal serum alt levels, immunostaining and liver biopsy which may not necessary for diagnosis but is helpful for grading the severity, staging, and damage of the disease.

Many hepatitis C patients do not manifest symptoms, but complaint of fatigue, mild discomfort or tenderness in the right upper quadrant, nausea, poor appetite, muscle and joint pains, along with marked increases in serum ALT and jaundice needed awareness by medical doctors of the importance of testing for acute hepatitis. Chronic hepatitis C is diagnosed when anti-HCV Is present and serum aminotransferase levels remain elevated for more than six months. Sometimes diagnosis is difficult in people who cannot produce anti-HCV, such as those who have another form of liver disease like alcoholism, iron overload or who are immunosuppressed or immunoincompetent. Some people with chronic hepatitis C have normal liver enzymes and some of them may show only very mild elevations of liver enzymes, which may not cause enough alarm for doctors to be concerned. In some cases hepatitis C is not detected until is too late and there is a need for a liver transplant.

The interval from the time someone gets the infection to time of irreversible scarring of the liver is 20 to 40 years. And once a patient develops cirrhosis or has severe liver disease, other symptoms manifest, including muscle weakness and wasting, itching, dark urine, fluid retention, abdominal swelling, ascites, ankle swelling, and jaundice. Physical exams with medical doctors are likely to be normal or show mild hepatomegaly or tenderness, with enlarged liver, spleen, vascular spiders, or palmar erythema and excoriations. Patients who develop cirrhosis or who have a severe disease may not have totally defined symptoms. It depends on the rate of disease progression.

Hepatitis D (infectious hepatitis, also called delta virus) is a small circular RNA virus. It only occurs in human in the presence of hepatitis B infection. In 90 percent of people, B and D is transmitted by blood and blood products, and most often in people sharing needles or intravenous drugs users. Hepatitis D and E are often called co-infection, side by side. Those two strains are much easier to diagnose.

Nowaday, all of us are at risk of developing liver-damaging disease either hepatitis A, B, C, and D. Some researchers say treatment remains complicated for people infected with those viruses. It is important to determine which virus is responsible, and the extent of damage to the liver to evaluate the severity of the illness.

All types of hepatitis warrant medical monitoring to prevent spread of the infection or development of cirrhosis and cancer. If not, once cancer starts in the liver which is often associated with prior Infection of hepatatis B and C virus. This requires medical attention and sometimes surgery to remove the primary tumor or a single metastasis or even a liver transplant.

Hepatitis E (enterically transmitted non-A non-B hepatitis or cecal-oral non-A non-B hepatitis)/(ET-NANBH). This virus is transmitted via the fecal-oral route. It may also spread from contaminated drinking water or foodborne transmission. The incubation period for hepatitis E varies from two to nine weeks. The disease usually is mild and resolves in two weeks. It is often seen in young to middle-aged adults (15 to 40 years old). Pregnant women mortality rate has been reported. Major water-bone epidemics have occurred in many countries. To date, no outbreak has occurred in the United States with the exception of Los Angeles in 1987. The best way to prevent this disease is through good sanitation and personal hygiene.

Hepatitis G (HGV virus infection) is a flavivirus related to hepatitis C virus (HCV). In 1995 and 1996 three viruses identified by investigators at Abbott Labs have been termed GB-A, GB-B and GB-C. GB-A and GB-B. Another group at Genelabs Technologies has identified and determined the complete genonlic sequence of the virus. These two studies show that persistent infection with HGV is common in the United States. Many studies suggest that novel flaviviruses may cause hepatitis in man and other primates. The precise role of HGV/

GB-C in human disease is under investigation by researchers. People with hepatitis C are likely at risk for GBV-C infection.

Lopez-Alcoroch et al. show that 15 percent of children with chronic hepatitis C or hepatitis B are infected with HGV, HGV co-infection does not appear to cause more severe liver disease. It was also identified in about 18 percent of patients with hepatitis C. HGV was detected in serum samples from patients in the United States, Australia, South America, and Europe.

In Japan, GBV-C/HGV implicating this virus as the cause of fulminant hepatitis. They also show HGV/HGBV-C infection is present in patients on hemodialysis. The influence of hepatitis G virus on the severity of liver disease is currently undergoing many pilot study all over the world.

Autoimmune hepatitis. Our own immune response is our defense against substances (antigens, pathogens). Its role is to seek out, identify and destroy those invading substances, which can cause disease or health problems. The stronger the immune system, the greater the immune response will be against disease-causing agents. But when the immune system becomes impaired, our own immune system attacks our cells. As in the case of autoimmune hepatitis, the patient's own immune system attacks the liver, causing inflammation and liver cell death. This condition resembles acute hepatitis with fever, jaundice, arthralgia, myalgia, and sometimes symptoms of mild to severe liver dysfunction. The disease usually occurs in 70 percent of women between the ages of 15 and 40. Any patients who have had a diagnosis of autoimmune hepatitis should have a liver biopsy with appropriate treatment. Most patients with autoimmune hepatitis respond to treatment.

Cirrhosis of the liver. It is a fact—the liver is the most important organ for detoxification. It performs many biological functions and many of the body's metabolic functions occur primarily in the liver as well as the metabolism of cholesterol and the conversion of proteins and fats into glucose. It's also where most drugs and toxins, including alcohol, are metabolized. When damage to liver cells from toxins, inflammation, metabolic derangements, and other causes occur, widespread nodules in the liver combined with fibrosis make the liver unable to perform its biochemical function. This can lead to to cirrhosis (irreversible scarring of the liver).

Patients with cirrhosis of the liver may have no clinical signs or symptoms, with the exception of fatigue. In advancing stage, patients complain of muscle weakness, poor appetite, nausea, weight loss, itching, dark urine, fluid retention, and abdominal swelling. Physical findings of cirrhosis included enlarge liver, enlarged spleen, jaundice, muscle wasting, excorlations, ascites, and ankle swelling.

Chronic liver disease, particularly cirrhosis, increases the risk of developing hepatocellular carcinoma. Most hepatocellular carcinomas are first suspected based on the results of CAT scans or ultrasound scans, and the definitive diagnosis of hepatocellular carcinoma is made by biopsy. Hepatocellular carcinoma is curable by surgery only if the tumor is small. But if the cancers become metastatic and spread from the organ like the colon, pancreas, lung, and breast, extensive treatment may be required. Your oncologist or medical cancer specialist doctor may offer chemotherapy. And there are many experimental therapies for metastatic cancers.

Hepatitis C is the leading cause of liver transplantation in the United States. This virus kills up to 10,000 Americans annually, and the death rate is expected to triple in the next two to three decades. According to the Centers for Disease Control and Prevention, only about 350,000 of those infected have been diagnosed. The best way to prevent hepatitis during early stages is to go to your medical doctor every year for a complete physical examination, including checking for any kind of hepatitis.

Some people become lifelong carriers of these viruses. If the virus is left untreated, itt becomes chronic and cirrhosis may result. Cirrhosis of the liver is irreversible but treatment of the underlying liver disease may slow or stop the progression. Chronic liver disease can lead to hepatocellular carcinomas to metastatic liver cancer and death.

Patient education is the key for prevention of the liver diseases and for those who would like to inform and learn about liver diseases should contact the National Digestive Diseases Information Clearinghouse (NDDIC), American Liver Foundation, Hepatitis Foundation International, National Cancer Institute, or American Cancer Society. The Internet is another source of information on this subject.

This bears repeating: It's not my intention for this book to take place of your medical doctors' advice. I encourage you to contact your medical doctor first.

But as a family practice healthcare practitioner, what impressed me most when I began to practice alternative medicine in 1985 is the way nutritional medicine was effective in patients with hepatitis. Nothing could be further from the truth. The liver is the detoxification center for the body, where all foods and beverages that we ingest pass through to be metabolized. Nutrition, diet, herbs, and others alternatives therapies will play an important role with hepatitis C patients. Here, I will be focus on alternative-preventive approach of the disease for those who want to be more informed about self care, integrated medicine that heals and puts the whole patient not the disease at the center of care.

ALCOHOL AND THE LIVER

Alcohol is toxic to the liver. It affects nearly every type of cell in the body, but primarily the central nervous system and the liver. In the brain, alcohol interacts with centers responsible for pleasure and others desirable sensations. For many people alcohol has dominated their thinking, emotions, and actions.

The fourth edition of the *Diagnostic and Statistical Manual of Mental Disorders (DSM-IV)* published by the American Psychiatric Association divides alcohol use disorders into alcohol dependence and alcohol abuse. Moderate drinking, at-risk drinking, alcohol abuse when the severity of the abuse affects their performance at school or on the job, while driving, and problems with the law. Often there is no clear line between problem drinking and alcoholism.

Some individuals continue to consume alcohol despite the knowledge that alcohol may pose significant problems in their social and personal relationships. Alcohol dependence occurs when there is evidence of tolerance and/or symptoms of withdrawal such as delirium tremens (DTs) or alcohol withdrawal seizures (rum fits) upon cessation of drinking. Unsuccessful Excessive intake of alcohol use can lead to acute and chronic liver disease, including cirrhosis and its complications liver cancer which is one of the ten leading causes of death in the United States. Social drinkers as well as heavy drinkers are at risk of liver disease.

Information about alcohol suggests that the hepatitis C virus has been isolated from patients with alcoholic liver disease and that may increase their risk of development of cirrhosis in an alcoholic. Alcohol can cause acute and chronic hepatitis. Alcoholic hepatitis is reversible if the patient stops drinking. If not, it can lead to liver scarring and cirrhosis in turn can lead to end-stage liver disease. The dangers of cirrhosis include jaundice, ascites, edema, bleeding esophageal varices, blood coagulation abnormalities, coma, and death. Therefore, the most important recommendation in the treatment of alcoholic liver disease is the total cessation of alcohol consumption.

Alcohol abusers require nutritional treatment with vitamins, especially thiamin. This may be a preventive medical step to correct the deficiencies and can reverse fatty liver and alcoholic hepatitis resulting from chronic alcohol abuse. Support groups such as Alcoholics Anonymous, Al-Anon, Alateen, and the National Clearinghouse for Alcohol and Drug Information may help with information about alcohol recovery programs.

Itching in liver disease. Itching in medical terms is known as pruritus. Today we still don't understand what causes itching and how scratching relieves it. This represents the biggest challenge in treating itching. Patients with primary biliary cirrhosis, primary sclerosing cholangitis, and hepatitis C frequently have itching, and it is a very difficult symptom for them and their medical doctors to manage.

Although researchers don't understand the nature of the substances that cause itch in liver disease, but they agree that accumulation of substances known as endogenous opioids (e.g., enkephalins) could be contribute to the itch secondary to liver disease. Others believe neurotransmitters pick up stimuli and transmit them on special areas of the brain, causing itching. Some theorize that other substances accumulate in the blood in liver disease, including bile acids, which may play a significant role in itching.

Always check your diet and what you eat; it may play an important role in liver disease patients who itch. Itching in liver disease can often be controlled with several medications. In some patients if itching does not respond well to treatment, your medical doctors will continue to look for other medications that may help minimize symptoms.

Reye's syndrome in liver disease. This is a type of encephalitis inflammation of the brain that affects the liver. It strikes children from ages 10 to 18 while they are recovering from a viral infection such as influenza or chicken pox. It is most commonly seen in children the age of five and 11 years, and most often occurs between December and March.

Reye's syndrome is a serious disease that requires immediate treatment. It's fatal in 25 percent of cases. A blood test is very important to determine the presence of liver damage and a blood sugar to monitor in children Reye's syndrome. Always check children for symptoms of vomiting, abnormal sleepiness or hyperactivity, and confusion. Convulsions and coma may occur as the disease progress. Aspirin should not be given to children with a viral infection, especially children with chicken pox and influenza. It has not been proven that aspirin causes or promotes Reye's syndrome in children.

Many prescribed drugs and over-the-counter medications destroy hundreds of thousand of liver cells and may have severe side effects on the liver. Tylenol (acetaminophen) alone is responsible for tens of thousands of liver poisonings each year, with hundreds of fatalities. It is not easy as one might imagine to provide conclusive evidence that drugs (medications) completely damage the liver. However, it has been clearly demonstrated both in the Physicians Desk Reference (PDR) and the Physician's Desk Reference for herbal medicines the precautions, interaction, and adverse reactions of every medications on some organ of the body, especially the liver. It is important for all readers to keep up-to-date on commonly prescribed pharmaceuticals, as well as certain over-the-counter products. Always check with a medical doctor if you are taking any medication.

Laboratory Test in Liver Disease: The term liver function tests (LFTs) is a popular term that asses the general stale of the liver and biliary system. There are many different testing methods to detect liver diseases. But the primary care physician must evaluate those results in combination with the history, physical examination, radiology studies, and biopsy to arrive at a reliable diagnosis. A recent study published in the *British Medical Journal* found that some patients with abnormal liver studies were not properly investigated, resulting interpretation, treatable and end results of chronic liver diseases. Therefore, it is important to distinguish between liver enzymes, liver function tests, and the meaning for patients which can help in the differential diagnosis and guide the diagnostic work-up of chronic liver disease.

LABORATORY TESTING PROCEDURES

Alamine aminotransferase (ALT). This is a liver function test that indicates liver cell damage. It is an enzyme produced by a major cell type in the liver, hepatocytes. All types of hepatitis (viral, autoimmune, alcoholic, drug induced, shock, drug toxicity, or toxins) cause hcpatocytes damage that can lead to elevations in the serum ALT activity. Elevated levels of AST, alkaline phosphate (ALP), and gammaglutamyl transpeptidase (GGTP) can present with one or both of two patterns. In chronic hepatitis or cirrhosis, the elevations of these enzymes may be minimal or moderate. The level of ALT in the blood is measured in clinical laboratory. ALT and AST are often used to monitor the cause of chronic hepatitis and the response to treatment.

Aspartate aminotransferase (AST). This is an enzyme similar to alamine aminotransferase that indicates liver cell damage. AST and ALT are located in liver cells. But AST is a more specific indicator of liver inflammation than AST. This enzyme is also produced in the muscle and causes elevation in other conditions, such as in early heart and hepatocellular disease. In alcoholic hepatitis and shock liver AST level may higher than elevation in the serum ALT level.

Alkaline phosphate. Alkaline phosphate is an enzyme produced in the bile ducts, intestine, kidney, placenta, and bone. Alkaline phosphate are elevated in a large number of disorders that affect the drainage of bile, such as gallstones or tumors blocking the common bile duct, or alcoholic liver disease or drug-induced hepatitis, blocking the flow of bile in smaller channels within the liver. When the serum alkaline phosphate are the main feature in liver disorders can be elevated in bile duct obstruction or bile duct injury as I said early such as patient with either cholestatic disease or infiltrate disease, neoplastic or granulomatous. It is also found in primary biliary cirrhosis or primary sclerosing cholangitis. It also can be elevated in bone disorders, carcinoma, head of the pancreas, ampula of vater, cholangiocarcinoma, pancreatitis, drugs, metastatic malignancy, sarcoidosis, tuberculosis, histoplasmosis, cytomegalovirus infection, and mononucleosis. Gamm aglutamyltranspeptidase (GGT) is utilized as a supplementary test to be sure that the elevation of alkaline phosphate is indeed come from the liver or the biliary tract.

Gain ma-glutamyltranspeptidase. GGT is an enzyme produced in the bile ducts that can be elevated in a large number of disorders, like alkaline phosphate, which affects the drainage of bile duct disease. GGT is a sensitive test and may be elevated in any liver disease and even normal individuals. There are many drugs, including alcohol, that cause elevation in GGT. In heavy drinkers even in the absence of liver damage or inflammation, GGT may increase. Elevations of GGT and alkaline phosphate suggest bile duct disease.

Bilirubin. This is the main bile pigment in humans. It is formed primarily from the breakdown product that results from the destruction of old blood cells called "heme" and others sources. Serum bilirubin is generally considered a true test of liver function (LFT). Elevation of the bilirubin causes the yellow discoloration of the skin and eyes called jaundice. Many liver diseases such as primary biliary cirrhosis or sclerosing cholangitis as well as conditions others than liver diseases can cause the serum bilirubin to be elevated.

Albumin. This is a major protein that circulates in the bloodstream. It is also only one of many proteins that are synthesized by the liver. Many liver diseases such as primary biliary cirrhosis or sclerosing cholangitis as well as well as conditions other than liver diseases can cause the serum bilirubin to be elevated. But when the liver has been chronically damaged, the albumin may be low. Also, malnutrition, some kidney diseases, and other rare conditions may cause low level albumin.

Platelet. Known as megakaryocytes, the smallest of the blood cells involved in clotting. Alow platelet count, decrease albumin, and prolonged prothrombin time are suggestive of decompensated liver disease. Patients with liver diseases, the platelet count decrease when cirrhosis has developed. Many others diseases also cause platelet count to be abnormal.

Prothrombin time (PT). This is a type of blood clotting test that is prolonged when the blood concentrations of some of the clotting factors made by the liver are low. In chronic liver diseases, the prothrombin time is usually not elevated until cirrhosis is present and the liver damage is fairly significant. Prothrombin time can also prolonged in non liver diseases, vitamin k deficiency, and some drugs like wartarin. The prothrombin time is also a useful test of liver function; it can measure the degree of liver dysfunction.

Serum protein electrophoresis. This is a major focus of the four types of serum proteins the serum electrophoresis are measured by: albumin, alpha-globulins, beta-globulins, and gamma-globulins. Serum protein electrophoresis is a very useful test in patients with liver diseases. In cirrhosis, the albumin decreased and gamma globulin elevated in some types of autoimmune hepatitis.

Iron in the liver diseases. The liver is the primary organ in the body that stores iron. Liver diseases have difficulty excreting iron from the body, especially in patients with hepatitis C and cirrhosis. Iron supplementation should be avoided in patients with liver diseases.

Sodium in the liver diseases. Ascites (abnormal accumulation of fluid in the abdomen) is one of the main complications of patients with advanced scarring of the liver (cirrhosis). A sodium (salt) restricted diet is very important.

Diagnostic tests in liver disorders. Many different test exist for HCV, anti-HCV (antibody to HCV), or HCV RNA. Current tests for anti-HCV are very sensitive. Some patients with hepatitis C test negative for anti-HCV (falsenegative reaction), and some patients who test positive are not infected (falsepositive reaction). False-positives and false-negatives can result when improper collection, handling, or storage occurs. It is not a routine screening test; there are patients who had resolved the infection but still test positive for anti-HCV. HCV RNA testing is a convenient test to determine a response to therapy.

Routine laboratory screening includes serum liver enzyme measurements, which should be done on routine physical examinations. An approach to interpreting liver enzymes elevations is very important, and it is helpful to divide patients with liver enzyme abnormalities into two categories: alkaline phosphate or transaminase spartase aminotransferase (AST) and alanine aminotransferasc (ALT) in order to determine what to do for the patient. If a patient is asymptomatic with no evidence of liver disease and only mild elevations in liver enzymes, he or she should have follow-up tests in one to three months. However, patients with liver enzymes that have remained high for more than six months are at risk for progressive liver diseases and need a complete re-evaluation by a physician who knows the entire case, and can interpret liver enzyme and liver function studies, and provide a reliable diagnosis.

PREGNANCY AND LIVER DISEASES

The liver is one of the largest and most important organs in the body. Pregnancy has little effect on a normal liver and causes no significant change in liver function. Certain markers of liver function may alter slightly during normal pregnancy. The protein albumin will decrease during pregnancy because of dilution of the expectant mother's blood.

Alkaline phosphate will increase during normal pregnancy because of the production of this marker by a normal placenta, and this small change does not indicate liver disease. It is important that all pregnant women be tested during the last two to three months of pregnancy for the presence of the hepatitis B and C virus. Even thus there are no recommendations to test women for hepatitis C and there is no specific preventive treatment available.

The babies of pregnant women who are infected with viral hepatitis may be born with it. Research indicates babies born to women carrying the hepatitis C virus are very unlikely to contract the viral hepatitis. It is recommended that all children should receive vaccination against hepatitis B since it is a preventable infection that may occur at any time.

Primary biliary cirrhosis, primary sclerosing cholangitis, and alcoholic liver diseases may impact pregnant women and their babies. Other liver disorders may have serious consequences for pregnant women and their babies, including introhepatic cholestasis of pregnancy (impaired bile flow), toxemia-related disease with the help syndrome, acute fatty liver pregnancy, toxemia or preeclampsia occurs late in pregnancy which includes: High blood pressure, kidney dysfunction, and the development of leg swelling or edema.

Ten percent of women with preeclampsia also develop blood clots and bleeding into the liver. In mild cases, liver function remains normal and in severe cases large parts of the liver may be destroyed. Toxemia or pre-eclampsia is life-threatening situation that can be occur at any time during pregnancy, especially for women at high risk. Many experts on liver diseases state that women who have had a successful liver transplant with good liver function can become pregnant. Only a few women who have had liver transplant and such women have successfully carried normal pregnancies. Although it cannot be guaranteed, the drugs used for immunosuppression after liver transplantation are thought to be safe for the developing baby.

Women with cirrhosis of the liver will have much more difficulty of become pregnant because of markedly decreased fertility. But, if they do become pregnant, they may be able to give birth to a healthy baby. They may, however, experience complications of liver failure during pregnancy. The baby is at high risk of premature delivery, spontaneous abortion, miscarriage, and stillbirth. In general, those children who are born, are generally healthy.

The liver and immune system. The liver is one of the organs that is very efficient at neutralizing or removing toxins. However, many people have deficiencies in their liver's function and in today's world the liver is overburdened by toxic chemicals that cause the liver to be clogged or even damaged or destroyed. The liver will need strong nutrients to detoxifying the body. The liver must constantly renew itself by replacing its 300 billion cells every six months. And because it is the primary filtering organ for our body, good health is impossible without a well-functioning liver.

Today liver disease has become an epidemic. In medical school, doctors are taught to diagnose and treat disease. They are trained to focus their attention entirely on the body. They think disease has nothing to do with immune system. In the past decade, medical researchers have made a profound shift of findings for safe and effective ways to enhance your immune system. In alternative medicine, we emphasize keeping the immune system balanced. When your immune system is unbalanced (upset), you are opening yourself to a whole range of illness, both acute and chronic, including cancer, viral syndromes (chronic fatigue syndrome, Epstein-Barr, herpes, HIV), parasitic infections, bacterial, fungal, or any other immune problems such as colds, flu, and allergies.

Although there is no scientific evidence indicating that liver disease is caused by a weak immune system, there are now hundreds of articles and studies show that when an inefficient immune system can't fight hard enough. Consequently, we get recurrent diseases affecting the whole body or diseases in organs such as kidneys, lungs, liver, or reproductive system. A healthy immune system means a healthy person.

The immune system is tremendously complex. What is important to understand when liver disease or others diseases occurs, our body's defender (the immune system) is unable to identify and destroy biological troublemakers. In my opinion, when your body discovers tissue damage or harmful invaders such as viruses, bacteria, and microorganisms, your immune system rushes to the rescue by dispatching powerful cells that attack and eliminate those invaders. The immune system has the ability to activate macrophage, which has the power to call the entire army—the reserves, even the special forces—including the thymus, a special kind of powerful white blood cells called t-cells or lymphocytes, antibodies, and macrophage (scavenger cells). Macrophage is the activator cells once he is activated he produce potent intercellular signaling molecules cytokines which activated T-cells, B-cells, monocytes and natural killer cells. As soon as your immune system sentries raise the alarm, the troops swing into action, assaulting any and all infectious-contaminated invaders, in a sense suffocating them in full force until they're totally eliminated.

Our bodies create 200,000 new immune cells and thousands of antibody molecules every seconds and engage in constant battle twenty-four hours without stopping with trillions of microorganisms in our body. It's essential that what we eat provides the body with the vital elements: amino acid, proteins, mineral and vitamin to build those millions of immune cells. It's no surprise immuno-nutrition plays a key role at every stage of the immune battle in alternative medicine.

Dr. Lius Poling, biochemist and two-time Nobel prize winner, has long been known for his research showing that vitamin C helps cure and prevent the common cold. Dr. Benjamin Siegel, a research pathologist at the University of Oregon in Portland, found in experiments the vitamin C not only increased immune responses, but also raised the blood level in interferon, one of the body's most potent germ-fighting chemicals.

Color in the Treatment of Liver Diseases

Understanding color's connection with human and spirit offers a key to maintaining physical health. Color has a powerful effect on the life of each one of us. Through time colors has been used by many different cultures, some administered as a form of therapy and some used as food, and we know that records back to the Egyptians time place value on sun colors. In China the emperor reserved the color gold for personal use and power. The Romans use red, the Greeks used greens and peacock blues. In early-ay medieval Christian art, every color had a mystic or symbolic meaning that the church gradually sanctioned. The Aztecs of ancient Mexico are said to have used irritating colors as devices of torture.

Many people write about colors, from Faber Birren's book, *Color, Survey in Words and Pictures,* from ancient mysticism to modern science, from Dr. Morton Walker and *The Power of Color,* from William G. Cooper and his research on the color in the form of light as part of the electromagnetic spectrum. William Benham Snow M.D., explains how blind people sense an object and color. Physicists Isaac Newton studied color spectral phenomena and developed the color wheel of three primary, secondary, tertiary and quaternary colors. Johann Wolfgang von Goethe in 1810 conducted research that remains unequalled even today on his work on color. Rudolph Steiner, the Austrian social philosopher, theorized that life radiates color and out of illness comes a new consciousness that re-establishes its balance in health and healing. Carole Jackson wrote *Color Me Beautiful,* about self-image color analysis. William J. Faber, D.O., medical director of the Milwaukee Pain Clinic and Metabolic Research Center in Milwaukee, Wisconsin, affirms that the mind and body are affected by color. Dr. Albert Einstein, physicist, opened our eyes to the complete spectrum of electromagnetic energy.

Certain colors used in hospitals to help patients for speedy recovery. The military also has used colors, as well as correctional institutions, schools, hotels, and businesses. Yet, for the most part, the western world continues to ignore the power of color in treating disease and their psychological and emotional effects on us and in our daily activities.

My general advice for preventing liver disorders in term of color is to avoid wearing certain colors that irritate and use color that has psychological and emotional effects to strengthen digestion and circulation. In my private practice I encourage patients who have liver disorders to use yellow and red. Color is the most noticeable component of the earth. Color is reflected light. Color has emotional appeal. Color has energy that affects us physiologically and psychologically. Whether we realize it or not, we can feel color and see it through our eyes and senses. Our psychological response to a color can affect us physically.

Yellow has many associations throughout history. It is the color of the universal communicator. For Egyptians, Chinese, and Greeks yellow became a symbol of power to sustain life. History says that the Chinese emperor owned exclusive rights to wear yellow and Chinese commoners were never allowed to wear it.

In the case of liver disorders, yellow has been associated with both function and repair damage. It helps in digestive aid, cleansing, and elimination in the liver, intestines, and skin. It energizes the alimentary tract, purifies the bloodstream, activates lymphatics, and depresses the spleen. It also acts as both a catarsis (purge) and a cathartic (laxative). Psychologically, yellow helps in maintaining confidence, indecision, concentration, and depression, and it also help releasing unwanted habits and emotion.

The most dramatic of all colors is red. Red has a strong character and is said to be an active and competitive color. The symbols of magic and ritual tend to be red. Some individuals will not be confident in their ceremonies if red not present. It gives them the sense of a strong leader who has the ability and energy to move the ceremony forward. Ceremony does not lie in what you are doing, but rather in how you are doing it and presenting it.

Females in red have a tendency to react quickly and emotionally, and not always objectively. Males in red like to be out in front, they want to show they are a leader. Most politicians enjoy wearing red to show that they are leaders. If you are choosing red, you have strength, courage, and conviction.

Red balances emotions and the mind; increases sex drive; activates blood circulation; stimulates the sensory nerves; and improves the senses of smell, sight, hearing, taste, and touch. Hemoglobin is made with red rays. Red rays produce heat that energizes the liver, the muscular system, and the left cerebral hemispheres. Because of anemia, constipation, and physical debilitation may seen with liver disorders, wearing red may have a profound psychological and emotional effects on your body. There are no undesirable effects in using color in our daily life. However, I cannot assume responsibility for the people who want to use color therapy in their daily life activities

For more information on color, I recommend John Ott's most current work *The International Journal of Biosocial Research.*

HEALING IN LIVER DISEASES

One of the best writers on dying Elizabeth Johnson with a foreword by Louise L. Hay state: "We are all, equally a part of the Eternal one. We are, in fact not only a part of the Eternal One, but, also, the Eternal One lives and expresses through us, as us. And life is a rich passage of Ideas, feelings, sights, sounds, experiences, and all forms of communication. Communication is the greatest power we possess. Without it, it would be impossible to communicate with the life force that each of us has within. The life force can be spirit, soul, God, source, force energy, bioenergy, cosmic energy, infinite mind, and many others.

Over the past 5,000 years, healing has been called many different names. The Chinese describe it as *chi* or *ki*; Indians call it *pran* or *prana*. Hippocrates called it *vis medicatrix naturae* (nature's life force). Christian religious often portray Jesus and other spiritual figures surrounded by fields of light. Christ himself called light the life-force. We see all religious speak of experiencing or seeing light.

Healing is an act of grace. Grace is a divine gift, a loving life force that enables us to communicate with our self a source of electromagnetic energy that flows through the body. Through grace we have the power of free will. A desire for purity and love between the soul and God. It occurs in purification when an individual integrates healing into his or her daily life experiences.

Without it, we feel alone. Praying by laying on hands is a relationship between your infinite mind (that is God) and you. I am not telling or forcing you to practice healing as a form of treatment but if you wish to learn self- healing, if you have any illness, whether it be psychological or physical, this experience will lead you on a journey of self-exploration and discovery. It can change your life from the inside out, as healing did for me since the death of my wife Alberte. Our attitude to healing determines how that healing will manifest itself. Action follows thought. Belief will create a sense of love in our hearts. We all have a very special way of healing our pain and disappointment. There are many books on the subject, if you are interested in studying this further.

COMPLEMENTARY/ALTERNATIVE APPROACHES IN LIVER DISORDERS

The use of complementary and alternatives medicine in liver diseases is rising dramatically. It's one of the reasons mainstream medicine is extremely slow to adopt any findings that do not originate in hospital or research facilities. Herbal medicine has reached a turning point. Not only is it fighting to be recognized as a science, but it has caught on like wildfire in this country because of the growing interest in the use of herbs among consumers, and because many studies confirm the safety and efficacy of herbal remedies. (Herb-drug interactions will be discussed later in this book.)

When I began practicing naturopathic medicine, I realized hepatitis A and C had become major public health issues in my community and since then I have conducted my own research. As I said previously, hepatitis A, which is transmitted in contaminated food and water, was most often seen in international travelers. Hepatitis B and C, blood borne diseases, resulted mostly from transfusions and needles. Hepatitis C, the virus, can remain in the body for 10 to 20, or even 30 years, slowly damaging the liver. If left unchecked by the time symptoms become evident, conventional treatment is not very effective.

Hepatitis C affects more than 4 million people in the United States and claims live of 10,000 people every year in this country. There is still no casual treatment available for virus hepatitis. In general practice, there is no drug on the market today, but the physicians will use standard treatment with interferon and other antiviral drugs which may costs up to 18,000 U.S. dollars per year. However, studies have shown that combining a complementary/alternative approach, including herbal and nutritional supplements, has been shown to have beneficial effects on the liver. And there are many physicians at the present who develop their own treatment protocol for patients suffering from a wide range of serious liver diseases.

HERBAL CONSIDERATIONS IN LIVER DISEASES

Many cultures rely chiefly on the special properties of herbs for promoting health. Today, the World Health Organization estimates two-thirds of the world population uses herbs as their primary medicine. Knowledge of herbal medicinal properties and their use has been recorded from pre-historic humans to the present time. It is wrong to think only pharmaceuticals agents can be very helpful in treating diseases. Chemicals are not only the answer. Herbs are considered food for the body. They have valuable source of vitamins, minerals, and amino acids.

The use of herbs in liver diseases, especially viral hepatitis, offers tissue support in regeneration, prevents necrosis of the liver cells, and aids in detoxification and elimination. They also support the liver's ability to inhibit viral reproduction. Research has shown the beneficial effects of herbs with antimicrobial, cholagogue, diaphoretic, laxative, and lymphatic actions of patient with liver disorders.

Some of the most potent liver regenerative and protective substances are as follows:

Milk thistle *(silybum maranum)*

Historically, this herb has been used in Europe as a liver tonic and currently is used in a whole range of liver and gall bladder conditions, including hepatitis and cirrhosis. It was also used in Germany for curing jaundice and biliary disease. Milk thistle was considered by many new and old world herbalists to be a liver protective agent in treatment of many liver diseases, particularly chronic hepatitis, cirrhosis, chemical, alcohol-induced fatty infiltration of the liver, and bile duct inflammation. The herb contains silymarin, a potent flavonolignans consisting chiefly of silibin, silidianin, and silichristine, which serve to improve, restore liver function, and prevent liver damage. Sylmarin prevents free radical from damage by acting as an antioxidant.

The herb has also been shown to be a potent inhibitor of this enzyme, thereby inhibiting the formation of damage leukotreines. Perhaps the most impressive action of sylimarin is the amazing restorative powers the herb's active ingredient, silymarin, has against liver damage. Several experimental and clinical studies on this herb revealing data about the herb's active ingredient and the reversal of toxic liver damage after the liver already been damaged. Milk thistle is known to treat several forms of cirrhosis, chronic hepatitis, and fatty infiltration of the liver, including alcohol- and chemical-induced fatty liver forms. The herbs can also indicate in the use of gall bladder conditions C (cholangitis) and subclinical cholestosis of pregnancy. It has been proved that milk thistle shortens the course of viral hepatitis and protects the liver against problems resulting from liver surgery. There is no drug on the market today, including interferon, that can protect the liver as well as the herb milk thistle. In addition, sylimarin a powerful free radical fighter and has ability to stimulate protein synthesis in the liver by increasing production of new cells to replace the damaged ones to allow production of new cells to replace the damaged ones. Also, it can boost levels of glutathione, improving the liver's detoxification processes.

Dandelion (*taraxacum officinale)*

Dandelion is known around the world by a variety of names. This nutritious, healing herb with a medicinal reputation dating back more than 1,000 years. Studies in humans and laboratory animals show that dandelion root enhances the flow of the bile, improves liver congestion, bile duct inflammation, hepatitis, gallstones, and jaundice. Dandelion root stimulates bile production, helps the body get rid of excess water produced by the liver, filtering toxins and waste from the bloodstream.

Chinese medicine and Ayurvedic medicine used this herb similarly. Two German studies suggest that dandelion stimulates the flow of bile, which helps digest fats. A 1983 study in Italy, by twelve patients with severe liver unbalance, symptoms of loss appetite, low energy and jaundice were treated with dandelion extract; eleven of the twelve patients showed drop in their blood cholesterol. Another study with dandelion extract was used to successfully treat hepatitis, swelling of the liver, jaundice and dyspepsia with deficient bile secretion.Dandelion has the ability to improve overall liver function. Dandelion is an herb of divination.

Angelica (*angelica sinensis)*

This Chinese herb, also known as *dang qui,* has been around since the dawn of history in medicine. Angelica has been used in medicine for thousand of years. Preliminary research reports from China suggest angelica increases red blood cell counts. It is also suggested that angelica increases the ability of blood clot and improves liver function in people suffering from cirrhosis and chronic hepatitis.

The Chinese still prescribe this herb for menstrual problems. Do not take this herb if you are pregnant as it can induce menstruation and abortion. Angelica is an herb of protection and healing. For infusion, use 1 tablespoon (tsp) of powered seeds or leaves per cup of boiling water, step 10 to 20 minutes

Licorice (*glycyrrhiza glabra*)

Licorice has been one of the most beneficial healing herbs around the world for thousand of years. It is one of the most extensively used and scientifically investigated herbal medicines. Chinese medicine has used licorice for centuries to treat liver problems. The herbs help control hepatitis and improve liver functions in cirrhosis patients. The major active component of licorice root is glycyrrhizin, also known as glycyrrhizic acid, and in Japan this herb is used in the treatment of chronic hepatitis and cirrhosis. It is an excellent anti-inflammatory herb.

Licorice is an herb that can cause retention of sodium and may raise blood pressure. Patients with history of hypertension, diabetes, glaucoma, stroke, kidney disease, heart disease, on currently pregnant or using digitalis preparations should be cautious regarding consumption of licorice. Licorice is on the FDA's safe herb list. Licorice is an herb of love, lust, and fidelity.

Gotu Kola (*centella asiatica* or *centella*)

This herb has been use as a medicine in India since prehistoric times. It is a traditional blood purifier, glandular tonic, and diuretic. The use of this extract in alcohol-induced cirrhosis, cirrhosis of unknown etiology, and chronic hepatitis has been reported. No effect was observed in the patients with chronic hepatitis, but in cirrhosis patients, improvement and regression of inflammatory infiltration was noted.

Gotu kola gained a reputation as a longevity promoter, attributed to LI Ching Yun, an ancient Chinese herbalist who used the blend regularly and lived a reported 256 years, surviving 23 wives. Gotu kola is an herb of meditation.

Berberine

This herb has been shown in several clinical studies to stimulate the secretion of bile choleretic effect and bilirubin, and it has also been shown to correct metabolic abnormalities in patient with liver cirrhosis.

Barbers *(barberis vulgaris)*

Oregon grape *(berberis aquifolium)*, goldthread *(coptis chinensis)*, and goldenseal *(hydrastis canadensis)* share similar indications and effects because of their high content of berberis alkaloids. The chief berberis alkaloid has a potent effect on liver problems. Overall barberry *(Berberis spp.)* stimulates the liver.

Garden Beet *(beta vulgaris)*

This is one of the best tonic drinks for the liver. Recommended intake is one glass each day.

Chevil uice *(anthriscus cereifolium)*

The liver is one of the major organs of the body assaulted by chemicals present in the food we eat, the beverages we drink, and the drugs we take. It is one of the organs of the body that shows evidence of abuse. Thankfully, the liver is capable of regenerating Itself. Chevil contains those components such as chlorophyl, mineral,salts, vitamins, and enzymes necessary for the regrowth transformation.

Tomato Juice From Garden Tomato *(lycopersicon esculentum)*

Restored the integrity of the liver to its original state of health. At the present time, there is a lot of research associated with the pigment that makes tomato red, the nutrient lycopene in the treatment of breast and prostate cancer.

Wheat Grass /Barley Grass (cereal grass)

These are rich in mineral salts and dark chlorophyll, which help to rejuvenate the liver by repairing some of the damage that has been done. Red current juice is good for liver jaundice.

Unripe Papaya

This fruit juice was used in India by Ayurvedic doctors for enlargements of the liver and spleen.

Radish Juice

This helps to break up the fat deposits in the liver, which cause liver to become enlarged because of sulphur amino acids contained in the juice. In Chinese medicine Schisandra berries promote healing of the liver can be made as tea bag and berry can also eaten whole.

String bean juice (*bean-phaseolus species*)

String bean and tomato and carrot juice, fresh canned and kyo-green from wakunaga will help to revive the liver or will assist this organ in recuparing from this type of abuse. One of the liver's functions is to remove toxic chemicals. Avoid processed foods, meats, and dairy products, as these add strain on the liver because they contain concentrated pollutants. Apples, carrots, citrus fruits, collard and turnip greens, parsley and fresh leafy greens, red beets and their tops, strawberries, summer squash, and tomatoes are considered.

Others Recommended Intriguing Possibility

Anise (*pampinella anisum*)

Since the time of the Pharaohs humans have found anise irresistible. Hippocrates, the father of medicine, found a more reasonable use for anise. He recommended this herb for helping to clear mucus from the respiratory system. One report shows that pimpiela anisum, anise, spurs the regeneration of liver cells in laboratory rats. This herb could be a value in treating hepatitis and cirrhosis in humans. For infusion, gently crush 1 teaspoon of anise seeds per cup of boiling water for 10 minutes and strain. Drink up to 3 cups a day.

Brussels Sprouts

Brussels sprouts are known to inhibit cancer, especially colon and stomach cancer.

Tumeric (Cucuna Longo)

They contain curcumin and other essential oils (turmerone, zingiberins). If you drink alcohol or take Tylenol (acetaminophen) regularly, you may risk liver damage. In this case, you may want to ask your licensed healthcare practitioner about using tumeric to protect your liver against damaging drugs. Tumeric has antifungal, antibacterial properties that offer protection and detoxification of the liver.

Yarrow (*achillea millefolium*)

This has been used in herbal healing for more than 2,500 years. A scientifically conducted trial in India showed yarrow help treat hepatitis. No animal or human studies back up this claim. However, two animal studies show yarrow protects the liver from toxic damage. If you have liver disease, add yarrow to standard therapies to protect the liver from toxic chemical damage. Yarrow is an herb of courage, power, and love.

Ginger (*zingiber officinale*)

This is now extensively cultivated throughout the tropical region of the world (e.g. southern Asia, India, China, Jamaica, Haiti, and Nigeria). Modern science has supported some of its traditional medicinal uses of varieties illnesses. One animal study shows that ginger shrinks liver tumors in experimental animals. Perhaps one day ginger may find its role in the treatment of cancer in humans. Ginger is an herb of money, success, love, and power.

Ginseng (*panax ginseng*) and Families

It's hard to explain the medicinal qualities of a plant that is popular all over the world. Ginseng protects the liver from effects of drugs, alcohol, and other toxic substances. In a pilot human study, ginseng improved liver function in 24 elderly people suffering from cirrhosis and liver damage from alcohol.

To drink, mix 1 teaspoon per half cup of water. Boil it, then simmer for 10 minutes. Drink up to 2 cups per day. Ginseng is an herb of love, healing, and protection.

St. John's Wort (*hypericum perforatum*)

This is a major star in the world of medicinal herbs. It has been used in herbal healing for more than 2,000 years. Hypericum, an extract of this herb, has been reported to be an antiviral against hepatitis B.

St. John's wort should be avoided by people taking antidepressants (MAO inhibitors and SSRIs such as Prozac). The asthma drug theophyllne (Theodur), the heart drug digoxin (Lanoxin), and migraine drugs in the triptin family Imitrex, Amerge and Maxalt). AIDS (protease inhibitors and non-nucleoside reverse transcriptase inhibitors) and anti-rejection drugs used by transplant patients.

St John's wort is one of the most popular herbs in managing mild to moderate depression. St. John's wort is an herb of divination, love, happiness, health, protection, and strength.

Shiitake and Rei-Shi Japanese Mushrooms

These are immune boosters and anti-cancer agents. They are thought to be beneficial in the protection of the liver against certain toxins.

Mushrooms *ganoderma lucidium* have been shown to have important medical benefit and have been used successfully in the treatment of viral hepatitis. Further research is needed.

It has been suggested that an herbal combination that includes licorice, peppermint, rose, tansy, and nettle can help stabilize liver cell membrane in experimental animals by protecting the animal from liver damage. Licorice (*glycyrrhiza glabra*) has a powerful healing action against liver disease, ulcers, or arthritis.

Green and Black Tea (*camellia sinensis*)

Tea has been the world's second most widely used herbal medicine for at least 3,000 years for treating many ailments. The Chinese claim tea can be used to treat hepatitis. Patients with chronic hepatitis have difficulty excreting iron from the body. Drinking green tea extract daily to lower toxic levels of iron, which can be very damaging to the liver.

Tea contains astringents tannins, and this astringent has some antiviral action. If you'd to like to incorporate tea in your treatment plan, do so only in consultation of your licensed healthcare practitioner. Teas are good for courage and strength.

Skull Cap (*scutellaria lateriflora*)

This herb is reputed to calm down people. Chinese physicians claim to have used this herb to treat people with hepatitis successfully. There are no others studies with skull cap, and this herb deserves further research and follow-up. Skull cap is an herb of fidelity, love, and peace.

Lecithin

Lecithin has a long history as a popular dietary supplement. Lecithin was first discovered in egg yolk (10 percent of a fresh yolk is lecithin). Today, the main commercial source of lecithin, including that used in injectable form, is the soybean. Lecithin is a product has been reported to be used in various illnesses ranging from cardiovascular disease, improving memory, increasing physical performance, and lowering risk of cancer.

Lecithin dietary supplement means different things to different people. In humans, tis role is crucial in the maintenance of cellular membrane fluidity of cells. Lecithin, which contains choline, can be taken in dosages of up to 1 to 2 teaspoons of granules daily to help improve liver function.

OTHERS HERBS SPECIFIED FOR THE LIVER

Alfalfa, black cohosh, black radish, barberry root, bahupatra bhuiamla, burdock root, cascara sagrada, cayenne, gentian, goldenseal, globe artichoke, indian almond, oregon grape root, skullcap, tamarind chicory, red clover, royal jelly, wild yam, and yellow dock have all been recommended.

THE ROLE OF NUTRITIONAL THERAPY IN THE TREATMENT OF LIVER DISEASE

The role of nutrition in the prevention and treatment of liver diseases has been extensively research and plays a major role in the treatment of liver diseases. It's important to include food in our daily life when we are faced with illness. The food we eat influences our nutritional status.

Hippocrates, the father of medicine emphasized nearly 2,500 years ago that food was the foundation of our health and happiness. Domage, in medical schools, "the Hippocrates oath was rewritten when he said to apply dietetic measures for the benefit of the sick according to my ability and judgment; keep them from harm and injustice anyone to measures for the benefit of the sick."

Today, many scientific studies show the benefits of food in humans. We see many people use food as their primary medicine. Herbs and food are full of pharmacological properties which can act as drug in the body. The common denominator underlying the effectiveness of herbs and food depends on the public how well natural product is good for them. But there is much recent evidence, particularly from physicians conducting research on herbs and food, that nutritional medicine might be an effective long-term therapeutic strategy for people with liver disorders and others diseases.

Books such as *The Food Pharmacy* by Jean Carpenter have demonstrated this. Almost everyone, at one time or another, has used natural remedies. Even most critics of using natural remedies to treat diseases uses herbs and foods everyday of their lives without realizing it.

A preventive approach of a daily multivitamin in the treatment of liver diseases, especially hepatitis, includes vitamin C (Ascorbic acid) with bioflavonoids (3,000 to 5,000 mg), and up to 10,000 mg in divided doses daily. Bring down to 500 mg.

Vitamin C assists the liver's detoxification efforts and is a powerful blood flow enhancer. One survey in the *British Medical Journal* links low tissue levels of vitamin C with environmentally induced disorders of the human liver. This is why vitamin C, a water-soluble vitamin, acts as a powerful antioxidant. It helps in the formation of liver bile and fighting viruses. The best source of vitamin C is fresh fruits and vegetables. This vitamin is also found in acerola berries,

Brussels Sprouts, Citrus Fruit, Currants, Parsley, and Rose Hips

Much different research was done with ascorbic acid for prophylaxis of viral hepatitis of administration high dose of this vitamin shows reduction in the duration of the illness with rapid recovery. Supplementation may be beneficial for prevention and treatment of hepatitis.

Vitamin A 10,000 to 25,000 IU Daily

Vitamin A (retinal, retinyl esters)/batacarotene is an anti-effective vitamin that acts as an immune booster. It helps cells reproduce normally and prevents invasion by disease-causing microorganisms. Vitamin A also helps to regulate and maintain a whole range of essential functions inside our bodies. In females who could become pregnant, it's recommended to take 10,000 IU (3,000 mcg) per day. And remember the liver has to convert beta carotene to vitamin A. Be careful of pill form of vitamin A. Beta carotene is a substance from plants that the body converts into vitamin A.

The best sources of vitamin A are from dark green, orange, yellow vegetables and fruits like carrots, sweet potatoes, apricots, pumpkins, and cantaloupes, and deep green leafy vegetables like spinach, dandelion greens, beer greens, chard, chicory, turnip greens, and kale. Also, one of the richest sources of vitamin A is beef. Beef liver is rich in the vitamin. Cod liver oil provides vitamin A. Individuals taking beta carotene for a long period of time, whenever taking vitamin E is advisable to take vitamin A may reduce the level of this vitamin. Some researchers said: in patient with cirrhosis vitamin A or beta carotene should not directly giving. Check-up the level of vitamin A first may be necessary.

Vitamin B Complex 100 mg Twice Daily

In the body, B vitamins function as coenzymes. Coenzymes are the keys that unlock an enzyme's effectiveness and allow it to take part in a biological reaction and they are essential for liver health. Therefore, daily supplementation of vitamins BI (500mg), B2(75mg),B5(1500mg),and B6(200mg) is highly recommended.

Vitamin B complex has been shown to be beneficial in patients with cirrhosis of the liver caused by excessive alcohol consumption; accidental, bacterial, or viral liver damage; exposure to toxic chemicals; or severe reactions to chemical drugs. Vitamin B3 (niacin) should be avoided in patients with cirrhosis.

Brewer's yeast is a natural source vitamin B. A large number of multiple vitamin/mineral products have B complex as part of their formula. If you are taking a multivitamin, there is no need to take a B complex.

Coenzymes Q 10 (Ubiquinone) 100 mg Daily

Not only does this counteract immunosuppression of viral infection, but they are also powerful antioxidant that are necessary for cellular energy production and respiration, providing support to all cells of the body and supportive of tissues that require a lot of energy, and protecting the body from free radicals. They also have blood flow enhancing properties and boost immunity for the cells of the body's natural defense system. More research is needed on this vitamin.

Folic Acid 400 to 1600 mcg Daily

Folic acid is necessary for red and white blood cell formation, maintaining the integrity of the nervous system, the conversion of homocysteine to methione, and the production of gastric HCL. It is essential for normal fetal neural development. It's also an antioxidant and blood flow enhancer for the liver.

Vegetables are the most important dietary source of folate (folic acid), for example: fresh cauliflower, broccoli, asparagus, cabbage, and Brussels sprouts.

Vitamin B6 (Pyridoxine) 50 mg Daily

Integretionalists believe vitamin B6 supplementation now has much value that this vitamin can prevent some of the side effects of a few prescription drugs, including oral contraceptives. Numerous reports indicate that pyridoxine can be beneficial in a wide range of apparently unrelated medical conditions.

Pyridoxine has attained the status of the master vitamin because it helps processing of amino acids, hemoglobin formation, nerve impulse transmissions, hormone synthesis, blood flow enhancer; boosts immunity; and is used for prevention and treatment of liver diseases. The best sources of pyridoxine are: brewer's yeast, meats, and whole grains.

Vitamin B12 (Cobalamin) 5000 mcg

Vitamin B12 a superstar in alternative medicine. Vitamin B12 is essential for normal liver function, has been shown to reduce recovery time, and has a dramatic effects in the treatment of various nerve-related disorder, among also others functions. B12 plays an important role in the maintenance of muscle tone in the gastrointestinal tract, the function of the nervous systems, the skin, the hair, and the liver.

Some members of the medical establishment believe B12 has had dramatic effects in the treatment of various diseases where conventional drugs and therapy has failed. Vitamin B12 may be very beneficial in the treatment of viral hepatitis.

Beef liver is the single best source of B12, as well as eggs, meat, dairy products, poultry, seaweed, spirulina, and fish such as mackerel, haddock, and salmon.

Vitamin B1 (Thiamine) 50 mg Daily

Every cell of the body requires this vitamin to form ATP, the fuel the body runs on. Studies show that vitamin B1 deficiency may complicate liver disease. Deficiency is most commonly found in alcoholics, those with bronchial cancer, breast cancer, eye problems, chronic liver diseases, people with malabsorption conditions, or those eating poor diet.

A thiamine deficiency may directly cause alcoholic cirrhosis, putting the patients at a greater risk for liver cell death. It is easy to correct. Giving them 20 milligrams of thiamine a year for 12 days brought their levels up to normal Clinica Chimica Acta

You can get enough of the nutrient from your diet in things like wheat germ, whole wheat, peas, beans, peanuts, fish, meat, brown rice, and seafood.

Zinc Sulfate 50 mg Daily

Zinc plays an important role in constipation, cell reproduction, and boosting immunity, and is essential for the normal storage and regulation of insulin and wound healing among other functions. Patients with cirrhosis of the liver benefit from 300 mcg (micrograms) daily.

Good sources of zinc are eggs, black-eyed peas, meat, seafood, oysters, tofu, and wheat germ.

Selenium 300 mcg Daily

Selenium, a trace mineral, has a powerful antioxidant properties, and has a vital importance in human metabolism, especially in the cellular membranes.

The most nuisible vitamin some said in the cell membranes are the sentinels of the cell. Selenium is known to contribute significantly in the soldier inside the cell by keeping the bad guys from entering the cell while he make sure the good guys in vitamins, minerals, and others nutrients).

Selenium is remarkable in slowing down the reproductive mechanisms and the replication of the C virus hepatitis. In addition, selenium provides protection against cancers and many diseases.

The best natural sources of selenium include broccoli, cabbage, celery, cucumbers, brewer's yeast, garlic, grains, fish, mushrooms, onions, organ meats, and radishes. (N.B.: Some naturalists do not give vitamin C with inorganic selenium at the same time and with the recommended dose toxicity is unlikely. But be aware of this high dose toxicity.)

Alpha Lipoic Acid 200 mg Daily

Alpha lipoic acid, or thioctic acid, is a potent antioxidant. It is involved in producing energy in muscles and directing calories into energy production.

Alpha lipoic acid is a meta-vitamin that plays a role in helping sustain normal blood sugar levels, supports the nervous system, and provides nutritional support for normal liver function. It has been shown to regenerate liver cells. Alpha lipoic acid protects the liver many ways. It can enter virtually all portions of cells to disarm free radicals unleased by the hepatitis C virus. It boosts glutathione levels to help in detoxification processes for allowing toxins free. There, by raising the glutathlone (major defenders of liver cells) levels, it can help prevent complications in cirrhosis or liver cancer. It restores energy to the liver by helping glucose into the cells, preventing regeneration of the severely damaged liver. Alpha lipoic acid could be the next important multivitamin.

For liver inflammation, saturated fatty acids, primrose oil as well as sulfur containing amino acids like: L-cysteine and L-methione 500 milligrams twice daily. And protein (free form amino acids) as directed on the labeled. Avoid animal protein.

(S-Adenosyl-Methione)

SAMe is an active form of the lipotropes choline and methionine used in Alzheimer's disease, severe depression, Parkinson's disease, and other degenerative brain disorders. Ongoing research found that it is effective at regenerating liver cells damaged by alcohol. It is a quite expensive and a cost-effective alternative to SAMe supplementation could increase the level of SAMe.

In the body is TMG (trimethylglycine) of dosage 500 mg tablets after meals, twice daily, or as directed by your licensed healthcare practitioner. Niacinamide protects the liver against alcohol-induced damage. Glutathione is a major defender of liver cells.

Glutamine

Glutamine may help reduce ammonia levels that build up in a damaged liver. Branch chained amino acids help in rebuilding damaged liver. L-leucine, L-isoleucine, L-valine, L-carnitine, L-arginine, Acetyl-L-carnitine, and N-acetylcysteine can enhance protein synthesis in the liver and muscle cells, and help facilitate liver regeneration.

Effect of silyrnarin on chemical functional, and morphological alterations of the liver. A double-blind controlled study.
Reference: Salmi HAS, Sama; Scand J Gastroenterology 1982 Jun; 1794 (4): 517–521.
Observations on the therapeutic value of intravenous B-12 in infective hepatitis. Reference: Jan. ASC, Mukerji DP., J. Indian Med. Assoc. 35: 502–505, 1960
Vitamin B-12 in the treatment of viral hepatitis
Reference: Campbell RE, Pruitt FW., Am J Med Sci 1952; 224–262
The effect of vitamin B-12 and folic acid in the treatment of viral hepatitis. Reference: Campbell RE, Prutt FW, Am J Med Sci 1955; 229:8
IP6 in the treatment of liver cancer. I. 1136 inhibits growth and reverses transformed phenotype in HepG2 human liver cancer cell line
Reference: Vucenik I, et al., Anticancer res 1998 Nov–Dec: 18 (6A):408–490
Vitamin C Prophylaxis for post-transfusion hepatitis
Reference: Pauling I. vitamin., Am J Clin Nutrition 1981; 34:1978
Chemo-prevention trial of human hepatitis with selenium supplementation Reference: Yus-Y, et al., Biol Trace Elem Res 1989; 20:15–22
Acute hepatitis treated with high doses of vit. C.
Reference: Calleja HB, Brooks RH.,) Int Acad Prev Med 1978; 5 (I) : 54
Intercellular glutatione as a possible direct blocker of HIV type I reverse transcription, glutathione antioxidant for the liver, necessary for the regulation of normal cellular growth and proliferation.
Reference: Kameoka M, et al., Aids hum retro viruses 1996 Nov 20; 12 170; 1635– 1638)
Treatment of hepatitis with infusions of ascorbic acid: comparison with other therapies
Reference: Baur H, Staub H.,AMA 156 (5 :565, 1954 (abstract)
Oral Zinc supplementation improves hepatic encephalopathy: results of a randomized controlled trial

Reference: Reading P, et al., Lancet 1984; 2:493
Vitamin E and cirrhotic muscle cramps
Reference: Konikoff F, et al., Int Med Sci 1991; 27:221–223
Zinc supplementation and amino acid-nitrogen metabolism in
patients with advanced cirrhosis
Reference: Marchesni G, et al., Hepatology 1996; 23:1084–1092
Is taurine effective for treatment of painful muscle cramps in liver
Cirrhosis? Reference: Marchesni G, et al., Am] gastroenterol 1993;
88:1466–1467
Cianidanol therapy for Hbe-antigen-positive chronic hepatitis. A
multicentre, double blind study. Reference: Susiki H et al., Liver
6:35, 1986
Vitamin C for prophylaxis of viral hepatitis B in transfused patients
Mrishige F, Murata A., Int Acad Prev Med 1978; (1):54
Aminoacid therapy of alcoholics hepatitis
Reference: Nasrallah SM, Galambos IT., Lancet 2:1276–1277. 1980
Use of polyunsaturated phosphatidyl choline in HbsAg negative
Chronic active hepatitis: results of prospective double-blind
controlled trial.
Reference: Jenkins P et aL,Liver 2:7–81, 1982
Clinical study of vitamin E status in patients with chronic hepatitis
Reference: Suzuki T, Kawase T, Harada T., Nippon Shokakibyo
Gakkai Zasshi 88(4): 1066 –1073, 1991
Enhancement of glucose disposal in patients with type 2 diabetes by
alpha-lipoic acid
Reference: Jacob S et al., Arzneimitelforschung 1995 Aug; 45(8):872–
874
Diet-induced changes in serum transaminase and triglyceride levels in
healthy adult men. Role of sucrose and excess calories.
Reference: Porikos KP, Van Italie TB., Am J Med 75:624, 1983

A branched-chain amino acid-supplemented diet in the treatment of
liver cirrhosis
Reference: Okita M, et al., Curr Ther Res 1984; 35:83

HOMEOPATHIC REMEDIES IN LIVER DISORDERS

Homeopathy is a natural therapy works with the body's own healing system, treating the person, not the disease. Given as a tiny remedy, it stimulates the body's natural response. The dosages are so tiny, they are extremely unlikely to have adverse effects. Homeopathy works with your symptoms to help cure illness, rather than suppressing them. Homeopathic is essentially the opposite of Western, or allopathic medicine. It treats disease with medicines that stop the symptoms instead of encouraging them. Samuel Hahneman called the will to health, or vital force, to effect self-cure *"simillia similibus curentur—let like be cured with like."*

Homeopathy has been used safely since 1810 when in the late eighteenth century, the German physician Samuel Hahnemann believed that the physician's job is to assist the body's natural healing mechanisms instead giving chemicals drugs to poison the body and override the natural mechanisms of the body. Since then, millions of people have been using homeopathy for the treatment of practically all types of illnesses.

Nux Vom, Acidum Fluor, Ratanhia 6c

Hamamelis 6c

Sepia 6c

Sulphur 6c

As directed on the label

This formula is necessary to stimulate the body's own defense, to generate resistance to the infection, to reduce the length and severity of the illness and to restore the patient to his state of health.

If jaundice (yellowish of the skin and whites in the eyes) is present as a result of liver disorder, this may be due to hepatitis:

Chamomilla 6c or Lycopodium 6c

As directed on the label and may be used in newborns.

Homeopathic treatment may be helpful for jaundice caused by hemolytic anemia.

One of the liver's functions is to remove useless toxic chemical. Tissue salts, three 6x tablets of natural sulfur dissolved under the tongue twice daily to aid liver function and the disposal of toxins.

GRANDMOTHER RECIPES

There is no doubt our ancestors, our grandmothers, deserve to be recognized. They spent a good part of their lives in forest looking for herbs to treat us. They keep what they learned in most precious part of their brain and passed it on to us. Today we benefit from their effort and they are my heroes.

In my city Tiburon, Haiti, 98 percent of people treat themselves with home remedies. Herbs are their primary medicines. Herbal cleansing is very important when the liver is in trouble.

How our grandmother learned what they did without going to school and having no high-technology laboratories is a mystery. I remember in summer 1993 I paid my late grandmother a visit. She looked at me and immediately said, "You need an herbal cleansing of liver and gallbladder flush" because of my belly (stomach) started to be enlarged. She told me that the liver performs more than 500 different tasks in the body. By detoxifying the liver, it has the power of rejuvenation. Even if 90 percent of the liver were to be removed, the remaining 10 percent could regenerate itself entirely. Why the liver and gallbladder flush is an important formula for restoring normal liver function.

The liver and gall bladder flush is accomplished by using castor oil packs placed over the liver area for several consecutive evenings at bedtime. Take one tablespoon of olive oil and pure lemon juice every morning before starting the detoxification program. Drink three glasses daily of distilled water with a half glass of apple cider vinegar, with fresh beet or carrot juice. Dink as much as apple or apple cider as your appetite will permit.

I encourage people to begin the flush on Monday and continue to Sunday noon, and also recommend a coffee enema three times a week with a day of apple juice fasting.

THE PURGATION FORMULA

Purgation is a formula that stimulates elimination through the bowel. Herbs used are aperients, laxatives, and purgatives.

The formula: First thing in the morning, use pungent herbs such as ginger, garlic, cayenne, nutmeg, or cloves for one to five days to help stimulate elimination through bowel. You may also have tincture of Oregon grape root (20 drops) in warm distilled water three times daily. Drink grapefruit or citrus juices for your evening meal. Do drink herbal teas and pure water to help your body eliminate the toxins that are being cleansed by the liver. Then go immediately to bed and lie on your right side with your right knee pulled up to close to your chest for 30 minutes. The next morning, one hour before breakfast, drink the juice of half a lemon in a cup of hot water; continue to do so each morning. On Saturday, after a week of flush, you should eat a normal lunch. And be sure to continue with your normal diet and any nutritional program that has been prescribed fro you by your healthcare practitioner.

Liver and Gallbladder Flush (Detoxification)
1 to 2 grapefruit or citrus fruits (1 to 2 oranges)
½ cup lemon juice or limes
½ cup unrefined olive oil
1 to 2 raw garlic cloves
pinch of cayenne pepper or freshly ground black pepper
(N.B.: If nausea or vomiting occurs when taking olive oil citrus juice, you need not to repeat the detoxification process again. But usually strong peppermint tea will help relieve nausea.)

Remember, the purgation formula should be avoided when there is abdominal pain, vomiting, and gastrointestinal bleeding. No food should be eaten before drinking the liver and gallbladder flush beverage. And you should abstain from eating for two to three hours following the flush.

Liver-Cleansing Tea Formula
2 parts dandelion herbs
1 part ginger root
1 part licorice root
1 part Oregon grape root
Mix the herbs together, simmer for 10 minutes in one pint of distilled water. Drink one-half cup three times daily.

Others recipes juice therapy is helpful for detoxifying, liver protective effect, cell production and oxidation in all of the body tissues: Drink carrot juice, red beet juice, green drink like spinach, celery fresh leafy greens, tomatoes and strawberries.

Although there is no specific diet that can prevent liver disorders, diet likely plays an important role in this process. Herbs, fruits, foods, and anything we ingest must pass through the liver. Good nutrition helps maintain healthy liver cells by strengthening the immune response against foreign substances (antigen, pathogens), which can cause disease. This gives the body a greater probability of increasing the body's resistance to infection and diseases.

Liver disorders contribute to malnutrition, reducing food-nutrient intake in the body. A good food contains a high content of vitamins and minerals, especially those with B vitamins for major defenders of liver cell. A low cholesterol diet is important in patients with hypertriglyceridemia.

It is recommended that all fats and dairy products be eliminated from the diet, as well as processed foods containing chemical additives, raw fish, shellfish, and sugar. The presence of fat in the liver may cause the liver to become enlarged, and it's advisable for patients with hepatitis C needs to maintain a normal weight with a low fat diet. Fat can cause liver function tests (LFTs) to be elevated.

Alcohol is a potent toxin to the liver. Avoid it or use in moderation. The recommendation is no more than one drink per day. But total avoidance of all alcohol is the best prevention of severe liver damage, cirrhosis, and a decreased lifespan. Take only medications prescribed by your physician as they put strain on the liver. Eating small meals is considered beneficial as well as cleansing fast. Protein is very important to build and maintain muscle mass and help in healing and repair.

Restriction of the diet of animal protein and staying on vegetarian diet is important to improve mental alertness. Liver is the primary organ in the body where iron is stored. Excess iron in the body can be a problem for the liver, especially in patients with chronic hepatitis C and cirrhosis, which means they have difficulty excreting iron from the body. Iron supplementation should be avoided with restriction of iron-rich foods: Any utensils with iron coated, nutrient supplement with iron, cereals fortified with iron, red meats (beef, pork, and veal), and liver. Not to mention also restriction of the diet of animal protein.

Many patients with liver diseases, especially hepatitis C and advanced stage cirrhosis, develop accumulation of fluid in the abdomen referred to as ascites. Sodium chloride (salt) restricted diets must be observed as well as nutrients to help eliminate the excess fluid in their body. Any patients on diuretics supplement potassium should be check and if low potassium supplementation is needed. Potassium deficiency may result if you are using diuretics, or if you are suffering from intestinal obstructions or inflammation. Always consult license healthcare practitioners if you suffer from abdominal pain of unknown origin, colitis, or constant diarrhea.

Any foods with high sodium should be avoided. Fast foods and red meats are high in sodium. There are many books available that list high sodium foods.

Drink distilled water, skim milk, and natural juices instead coffee and soft drinks. A tincture of 20 drops of Oregon grape root in warm distilled water should be taken three times daily. As always, drink ½ teaspoon of lemon juice and ½ teaspoon of cod liver oil each morning help to detoxify the hepatotoxins and help cleanse and rejuvenate the liver.

Thomas Edison stated: "The doctor of the future will give no medicine, but will interest his patients in the care of the human frame, in diet, and in the cause of prevention of disease." At the Institute of Natural Medicine, our approach is different. We combine Western medicine, complementary medicine, holistic medicine, and natural medicine to form one medicine that heals and puts the whole patient, not just the disease, at the center of care. We call it integrated medicine. This practical integrates approach allows us to combine Western medicine's diagnostic tests with our herbal and nutritional program.

Here is an example of recovery from high liver enzyme in alternative medicine:

Chief complaint text: Abdominal swelling from free fluids with general fatigue, loss appetite, decrease energy, and lethargy; enlarged liver was discovered upon physical examination in 1996.

History of present illness: A 64-year-old black female from the West Indies accompanied by her daughter to the Brooklyn natural center, claiming she was diagnosed with hepatitis C in 1994 following routine blood work. At that time her illness was classified as end-stage cirrhosis and she was advised there was nothing they can do at the hospital for her. According to her daughter, liver transplant was not even considered. The patient also had a history of hypertension and varicose vein legs bilaterally for the past 10 years. No psychiatry history. She believes she has allergy to some food derivatives, but oherwise she has no known allergies.

Substances use: Tobacco six to 10 cigars per daughter. Patient quit 10 years ago. No drug or alcohol use.

Family/social history: Patient grew up in a big city in the West Indies where her parents remain. As young girl she worked in a bakery baking bread for many years. While in the West Indies, she had been in two marriages at a young age. Her first marriage involved an incident of domestic abuse where she was badly beaten. Her second marriage involved an incident of domestic abuse again where the husband had three to four wives together. She has lived in the United States since 1990 with her daughter. She denies any family history of psychiatric disorders.

Physical exam: Her vital signs were stable. Her general appearance was thin, affect, and in no acute distress. On approach she appeared sad and hopeless about her illness.

She was AAO x 3, had dry mouth and lips, positive tenderness upon palpation of the abdomen, with enlarged belly, back pain upon palpation with 3+ piting edema and no cyanosis. The rest of the physical exam was unremarkable. Liver enzymes remained elevated and the disease was believed to be progressing because of a drop in her platelet count.

Her long-term goal was to return to the hospital, maintaining treatment and compliance with her medications and at the same time establishing therapeutic relationships between allopathic and alternative medicine. She decided to use natural therapies to treat her condition, and was started on some botanicals to support the liver, along with lipotropic factors. Liver enzymes decreased minimally but no change in platelet count was noted. After three months of alternative treatment, she was given intravenous vitamin C with others nutritional supplements, alternating with intravenous hydrogen peroxide for one time only. Seven days after this initial treatment, major autohemotherapy with ozone was begun and continued for 30 days.

Working diagnosis: Chronic hepatitis C with stage cirrhosis and hypertension with varicose veins problems.

Laboratory studies shows: Her liver enzyme on 3/21/96 LDH 646

SGPT / ALT 880 SGOT /AST 340

Slowly, month by month liver enzymes decrease and within six months reduced by:

ALT 32 AST 41 LDH 184

Combining allopathic medicine's diagnostic tests with our integrated nutritional herbal protocol, we have been able to monitor, to evaluate the progress of her with many other patients of their recovery and provide them a speedy recovery from this serious incurable disease hepatitis C (HCV). Follow-up clinical examination and appropriate blood work revealed the patient was free of any hepatitis C virus, and she has continued to remain healthy, with normal energy levels. At her six month follow-up exam, she remained exuberant and healthy.

At the Brooklyn Natural Center, we assess the patient's complete physical and mental make-up and determine whether the problem is from an inside or outside source. We also rely on traditional Chinese medicine of a combination of signs and symptoms patterns: retention of damp heat, invasion of the spleen by damp, stagnation of liver chi, and disharmony between the spleen and stomach. They must be visual, audient, and subjective. Physical appearance is assessed, the tongue is examined, and the character of the pulse is determined, along with other observations. If necessary a hepatitis profile, including SMA 18 with liver enzymes and a complete blood count (CBC).

We look for the following symptoms of poor liver function:

- Fatigue
- Irritability
- Depression
- Poor concentration
- Allergies
- Post menstrual syndrome (PMS)
- Menopausal difficulties
- Headache
- Indigestion
- Hypoglycemia
- Cirrhosis
- Liver damage
- Cancer

After the complete evaluation, we determine if liver function is poor, an indication that the liver energy is impaired. The treatment principle is clear in correcting the problem: clear heat, damp elimination, invigoration of the spleen, soothing of the liver, and regulating of the chi.

We design a personalized treatment plan to stimulate your body's own healing power. The first step of the first visit is an intake interview of all necessary information needed to make a complete evaluation. The intake information is similar to those of a conventional medical intake. But some additional questions are asked on health history, behaviors, both physical and emotional health, diet, and lifestyle. This is followed with a physical examination and appropriate laboratory testing, if necessary which is an important tool. It is important also to inform us about any therapy you are currently using, including any dietary supplements. This is enables us to learn about the factors affecting your health.

The second step is the review of findings and interpretation of the lab testing, physical exam, and the initial visit to help establish treatments protocols. A follow-up visit is necessary in three to six weeks to help ensure the result of a safe and coordinated course of care. The goal of the center is not only to help improve your health now, but to prevent future illnesses, helping your body grow stronger and resist disease more effectively. Alternative treatment at the center is always individualized with references to scientific studies that provide justification for integrated-alternative therapies.

There are conventional medical treatments available for hepatitis C and others liver disorders, but some people also try complementary-alternative medicine. Even thus alternative medicine has not yet been proven safe and effective for treating hepatitis C and liver disorders. CAM (complementary-alternative medicine) has many treatments for people with hepatitis C and liver disorders.

At the center, we combine what we consider the most effective and useful nutrients that may be helpful in supporting the liver, including:

- Royal jelly
- IP6 (inositol hexaphosphate)
- The immune support
- The E and I support
- Betaine HCL pepsin
- Probiotic fomula
- Vitamin A 25,00 IU
- Calcium 100 mg/Magnesium 500 mg/ Vitamin D 400 IU/ Boron 3 mg/Zinc 4 mg
- Ultra flush/internal cleanser
- Aerobic 07 liquids
- Milk thistle sylmarin extract
- Four herbs formula
- Papaya enzymes
- Jiggao pill formula
- Jangmeiling formula

- Ganfuning capsules formula
- China gold formula
- HEP-forte, hepatic-lipotropic nutritional support

Royal Jelly
Dosage: One capsule before meal, twice daily. A powerful biological product, rich in proteins and vitamins. For hepatitis, efficacious in restoring the function of the stomach, malnutrition, loss of body weight, and general weakness.

IP6 (inositol hexaphosphate)
Known as phytic acid by Pure Encapsulation, Inc. Dosage: Two to four capsules per day, in divided doses, between meals. It is a natural defense system support and a cellular function support shown to nutritional promote prostate, breast, colon, and liver cell health.

The Immune System Support
By the Brooklyn Natural Center, Inc. Dosage: Two capsules with a meal daily as a dietary supplement to support detoxification and immune system functions. ISS contains 20 vital synergistic nutrients including the key antioxidants A,C,E, and selenium, which supports all aspects of the body's natural cell defense system.

The E and I support
By the Brooklyn Natural Center, Inc. Dosage: As a dietary supplement, dissolve one tablet in mouth three times daily. A dimethylglycine supplement to support endurance and immune system function found In the cells of all plants and animals; has been found effective In enhancing the body's immune system.

Setaine HCI Pepsin

By Pure Encapsulation, Inc. Dosage: One capsule with each meal daily. A very important formula for proper digestion of food and proper absorption of nutrients and needed fro calcium uptake.

Probiotic Formula

By the Brooklyn Natural Center, Inc. Dosage: As a dietary supplement, take one to two vegetable capsules daily. To maintain healthy intestinal flora, necessary for liver impaired.

Vitantin A 25,000 IU

By the Naturally Vitamin, Inc. Dosage: Start with 50,000 IU daily for four weeks, then decreases by 25,000 IU daily. Vitamin A on emulsion form, essential nutrient for wide range of nutritional support for the entire body and for the body's defense systems.

Calcium 1000mg/Magnesium 500 mg/Vitamin D 400 IU/Boron 3 mg/Zinc 4mg

By the Brooklyn Natural Center, Inc. Dosage: As a dietary supplement take four tablets daily. This formula is essential for blood clotting, which is a problem in liver diseases.

Ultra Flush/ Internal Cleanser

By the Vitamin Power. Dosage: As dietary supplement, add one a half tablespoons (approximately 11.25 gm) cleanser to an 8 ounce glass of juice. Mix well and drink immediately. Follow with an additional 8 ounces glass of juice or water. For optimum effectiveness, drink 30 minutes before each meal. Ultra flush/ internal cleanser is a natural fiber supplement with herbs, soy protein, lecithin and super foods nutrients.

Aerobic 07 Liquids

By Aerobic Life Industries, Inc. Dosage: Treat and/ or freshen water with six to eight drops per gallon. For higher oxygen concentration, add six drops per 8-ounce glass of water. Aerobic 07 is a liquid solution of stabilized oxygen with buffers and electrolytes. An effective dietary supplement to help prompts the formation of white blood cells, which can help the body maintain good health.

Milk Thistle Sylmarin Extract (*silybum marianum)*

By Pure Encapsulation. Sylibum marianm contains one of the potent liver protecting substances known. Research shows that silymarin protects intact liver cells and stimulates protein synthesis. Dosage: Two to three capsules per day, in divided doses between meals.

4 Herbs Formula 4:1 Extract, 450 mg

By Herbal Healer Academy Inc. A dietary supplement with burdoc root, sheep sossel, slippery elm bark, turkey rhubarb may benefit by adding dandelion herbs to the formula will benefit people with hepatitis C. Dosage: One capsule three times daily with lukewarm water

Papaya Enzymes

By Brooklyn Natural Center, Inc. Dosage: Three tablets daily. Papaya enzyme works on undigested food remaining in the colon and reduces inflammation.

Jiggao Pill Formula

By Yulin Drug Manufactory in China. JGP is an effective remedy for curing all kinds of hepatitis and others inflammation diseases, particularly for curing jaundice type hepatitis and the yellowness of the skin. Method of taking: Three times a day for adults, four pills a time; for children, reduce that to half. Take with lukewarm water.

By Guabgzhon Guang Hua Pharmaceutical Co. in China.

A specific formula for acute, chronic, and prolonged hepatitis with excessive glutamic pyruvic transminase in the serum caused by other diseases (including other types of liver diseases). Dosage: Adults, two to three capsules, three times daily

Gan Fu Ning Capsules formula

By Guangzhou. From a plant, rhodomyrtus, tomentosa's dried root. Gan Fu Ning has been used in China in the treatment of anicteric virus hepatitis, infectious hepatitis, or acute icteric hepatitis, and especially chronic hepatitis. Each capsule contains 200 mg of rhodomyrtus tomentosa's dried root extract. Dosage and administration: For adults, one capsule, three times daily. Take continuously for one to two months after recovery of hepatitis for strengthening efficacy.

China Gold formula

By Aerobic Life Industries, Inc. Suggested directions: Shake before using. Drink ½ to 1 ounce (15 to 30 ml) twice daily, preferably before morning and evening meals. China gold is a liquid herbal formula contains 36 botanical herbs, flowers, mushrooms, fruit, root, and bark of selected Chinese botanicals plants which tonifies the lungs, stomach, heart, liver, and kidneys, strengthens the spleen, sinews, bones, nourishes blood, benefits the mind, and generates fluids.

Hep-Forte Formula

By Naturally Vitamin, Inc. MA Hepatic-Lipotropic Nutritional Support to maintain healthy liver functions. For use as a dietary adjuvant for persons receiving professional care for liver malnutrition. The recommend dosage is one softgel six times daily, as directed by a healthcare professional.

Although our base protocol is mostly supplements recommendation of herbal, multivitamins and Chinese herbs possible with recommend acupuncture and acupressure to soothing the liver and regulating of chi. Chi, or life energy, circulates through the body, mainly along the acupuncture meridians. Chi disease results from imbalance or stagnation of chi in the body. In hepatitis poor liver function occurs as an indication that the liver needs to cleanse and detoxify.

The treatment plan often includes cleansing, detoxifying, and elimination of toxins that can hasten the destruction of the liver.

Dietary recommendations including eating organic food whenever possible, eating a high fiber diet, and drinking plenty of pure filtered water to help flush out toxins. Recommended lifestyle changes include avoiding alcohol, caffeine, smoking, and any chemical drugs.

USEFUL RECOMMENDATIONS

Liver is the body's fuel filter performs many functions essential to life and the quality of virtually every body function depends on the liver. When waste accumulation cause lever become too congested, a potent liver cleanser is necessary such as foods like: fresh green vegetables, dandelion greens, beets, carrots, mustard greens, watercress, garlic, ginger, arugula, grape fruit, kale, endive, collards greens, lemons, limes, and parsley. Those herbs are helpful for stimulate the flow of bile, which naturally cleanses the liver and improves digestive function. These herbs have antimicrobial and antiseptic properties that help to clear the digestive tract.

Beet green herbs are very important in helping the liver to stimulate bile flow and cleansing. The liver is designed to protect our bodies from harmful substances, pesticides, solvents, toxic chemicals, drugs, and food additives. A high protein diet is vital for liver health. The best proteins are from brewer's yeasts, sesame seed, sprouts seeds and grains, raw goat's milk, raw nuts like almonds, and raw cottage cheeses. Some of those nutrients are rich in B vitamins and have high contents of methione, calcium, and unsaturated oils.

Avoid all forms of salt, sugar, irritating seasonings, white flour products, commercials cereals, all processed or artificial, canned, and refined foods. Avoid all chemical additives in foods and poisons in air, water and environment. Avoid alcohol, soft drink, tobacco, fatty and fried foods, rancid oils. Avoid raw fish, shellfish, and animal proteins. Don't exercise too soon after eating. Avoid bedtime snacks and eat meals at least three to four hours before lying down and elevate the head of your bed at least 45 degrees this can increase abdominal pressure because it is important for proper indigestion. Sitting or standing instead lying down helps keep the stomach acids in the stomach if you have heartburn.

Use honey, low sugar diet, skim milk, red beets and their tops, red beet juice or beet powder with cucumber, garlic, and summer squash.

Eating small, frequent meals lightens the liver's load. Distilled water, natural herbal, and juices should be used. If jaundice is present, the patient should be put on a one week juice fast. Drinking a glass of carrot juice plus 8 ounces of either apple, celery, beet, citrus, cucumber, or grape juice twice daily is also advised. At the same time lots of exercise, fresh air, and plenty of rest. Many drugs are liver toxicity. Under no circumstances do not take any drugs prescribed by your license physician. Try to avoid constipation and straining during bowel movements. If this happens, it is necessary to use the following liver cleansing method: Mix 20 ounces of fresh lemon juice with 20 ounces of olive oil. For two nights, take 1 cup of this mixture. On the third evening, take a double dose (40 ounces of each). On the following morning, take catnip tea enemas and 1/4 teaspoon lobelia tincture every four hours. (Lobelia should not be taken internally on an ongoing basis.) I will prefer instead lobelia, added one cup freshly brewed coffee. The coffee enemas should be retained for as long as possible up to 20 minutes. Repeat the coffee enema in the evening.

Use retention coffee enemas every twice a week. You may also use chlorophyll enemas three times a week—at least one pint and retain for 20 minutes. Castor oil packs over the liver area during night for 30 minutes to two hours is also recommended. Make sure to get plenty of bed rest.

PARENTAL NUTRITION IN INTEGRATED/ ALTERNATIVE MEDICINE AND LIVER DISEASES

Total parenteral nutrition was used successfully as a valuable clinical technique more than 25 years ago. Today, with the knowledge of micro nutrients and molecular biological revolution, parenteral nutrition has been a very useful benefit in the management of patients with various illnesses. Many studies have been published on the efficacy of nutrition therapies for the treatment of hepatitis. Although research in alternative medicine is limited, there have been a few recent studies, such as that conducted at the Bastyr University Office of the Alternative Medicine at the Institutes of Health, and others which had as their goal to develop nutritional therapies to treat illness.

There was evidence in the medical literature that intravenous parenteral nutrition used in optimum doses in hepatitis patients.

CHELATION THERAPY IN LIVER DISEASES

Chelation therapy is a process of removing heavy metallic ions from the human body by injecting EDTA (ethylene diamine tetracetic acid, also called eidetic acid) into the veins. It is administered intravenously and is often given with multivitamin and mineral supplementation and the solution may contain others nutritional supplements at the practitioners discretion. EDTA is attaches itself to harmful plaque, lead, and other heavy metals, and extracts calcium from cells in the walls of the arteries, which are found in many advanced atherosclerotic plaques.

Chelation therapy in the mid-1900s originally was found to be effective in treating heavy-metal poisoning. In the early 1950s, researchers of EDTA found that he is effective in removing metastatic calcium deposits from the human body. Since, then there is a large number of clinical observations on EDTA, but many of them have not been published and no supportive evidence of the effectiveness of chelation therapy. Now a growing numbers of physician of physicians have recommended it as an effective option alternative to angioplasty or bypass surgery in treating coronary artery disease. Advocates of chelation therapy claim that the treatment is safe, economical, and effective therapy for many other diseases, including qngina pectoris, diabetic gangrene, lupus, psoriasis, thrombophlebitis, scleroderma, hypoglycemia, lead toxicity, cerebral degeneration, thyroid disorders, multiple sclerosis, muscular dystrophy, high cholesterol, hypercalcemia, hardening of the arteries, cancer, and Alzheimer's disease.

Chelation therapy is controversial and research does not yet support this treatment as important method of treatment for illness, including liver diseases, other than for removal of heavy metal poisoning. Many patients involved in chelation therapy are advised to make changes in their diet and exercise, take dietary supplements, and participate in a stress reduction program. If you are considering chelation therapy, contact the American College for Advancement in Medicine, 23121 Verdugo Drive, Suite 204 Laguna Hills, CA 92653; or the American Board of Chelation Therapy 1407-B North Wells Street, Chicago, IL 60610.

HYDROGEN PEROXIDE THERAPY IN LIVER DISEASES

Hydrogen peroxide (H202) normally name is hydrogen dioxide of a colorless liquid of blue in thick layers odorless liquid that mixes easily with water. [SEE QUERY ON ORIGINAL MANUSCRIPT, PAGE 124]

Hydrogen peroxide breaks down into oxygen and water:

Catalase or

H202 > > > > 02 + H2O

Peroxidase

Nearly most of the hydrogen peroxide found in traces in natures, rain, and snow. The solution is available in several concentrations. The 3 percent concentration used for skin wounds or mouth ulcers. The 6 percent is used to bleach hair and the 35 percent is used as a nontoxic disinfectant by the food industry.

The clinical benefit is the use of intravenous administration of hydrogen peroxide as oxidative detoxification, which relieves allergic reactions and helps the immune system by stimulating production of white blood cells, including T-helper cells. It also benefits patient with pneumonia, inflammatory joints, rashes, fungal conditions, and chronic diseases. This may be because of the oxidation of some foreign substances in the blood. Initial results are very promising on the treatment of cancer, emphysema, AIDs, and other diseases.

There's no doubt hydrogen peroxide will put extra oxygen in your blood. A body with more oxygen is more flexible and able to have a strong immune system, which is an important part of staying healthy and avoiding serious illness.

Intravenous hydrogen peroxide can be beneficial to diseases such as diabetes, hypertension, Epstein-Barr virus, Parkinson's, emphysema, arthritis, asthma, ulcers, candida, cancer, HIV, lupus erythematosis, multiple sclerosis, cardiovascular diseases, herpes zoster and simplex, headaches, bacteria, fungus, parasites, viruses, and tumors. Many studies have shown the benefit of H202 in certain diseases.

Some practitioners in intravenous hydrogen therapy suggest using hydrogen peroxide 2.0 cc with normal saline 200 ml over a period of with hours with careful monitoring of the patient. Or hydrogen peroxide 2.5 cc, sodium bicarbonate 0.75 cc, with D5W (dextrose with water) 250 ml; vitamin B12 (cyanocobalamin) 3.0 cc may be added.

Now hydrogen peroxide can be taken orally at low doses of concentration and can be purchased in natural food stores. It can also be used for people with psoriasis, stiff joints, rashes, and fungal infections.

RECIPES

Take a bath of 1 pint of 35 percent food-grade hydrogen peroxide in a tub filled with warm water and soak for 20 minutes. It can be repeated one to three times per week until the infection is clear. For more information, contact IBOM, Ozome and Peroxide Referrals, P. O. Box 13205-OT Oklahoma City, OK 73113; or ICMA, P.O. Box 61767 Dallas, TX 75261.

MAGNETIC THERAPY IN LIVER DISEASES

Magnetic therapy dates as far back as from our early ancestors from ancient Egypt, China, India, and Greece. Magnets have been used by Chinese healers as early as 200 B.C., long before the existence of any known writings and system of medicine develops. Chinese healers were able to use magnetic lodestones on the body to correct unhealthy imbalances in the flow of this internal strength chi, or energy.

The ancient Chinese medical text book known as *The Yellow Emperor's Book of Internal Medicine,* the earliest written record of medicine, dates back to 2000 B.C. It describes magnetic therapy as well as imbalances corrected by means of acupuncture, moxibustion (heat), and application of magnetic stones as compasses. The ancient religious scriptures of the Hindus, believed to be 4000 years old, known as the Vedas, mention the treatment of disease with asthmana and siktavati, "instruments of stone."

The word magnet comes from the young Greek shepherd named Magnes Lithos, or Stone from Magnesia, in a region called Magnesia, rich in magnetic stones, which later became magneta in Latin. From ancient Greece philosophers and mathematicians to Egyptian physicians, the Chinese magnetism, electricity, and energy have a strong influence on our lives today. In the United States, interest in magnetic therapy began in the 1990s, as several therapists offered testimony of some benefits that magnetic therapy claims to provide include: pain relief, reduction of swelling, improve tissue alkalinization, more restful sleep increased tissue oxygenation, relief of stress, increased levels of cellular oxygen, improve circulation, and anti-effective activity.

In the United States, at the present time, magnet therapist are not allowed to make claims, even though some double-blind studies have proven to be effective in pain relief and completely safe. Over the past 155 years, scientists have been studying the decline of magnetic field and the effects it has on human health, and more modern contributions on medical knowledge of electrical and magnetic energy were made of successful treatment of a variety of diseases. There are no harmful exposure levels of the natural energy source produced by magnets, yet it is not widely accepted as an official method of pain relief.

There are no preparations for using magnetic therapy other than purchasing the products. There's a lot of benefit reported by individuals using magnet as a form of therapy as necklaces and bracelets; knee, back, shoulder and wrists braces; mattress pads, gloves, shoe inserts, and more. If you have liver disorders, it is worth it to try magnet therapy.

Magnet therapy is self-administering. At the present time there is no training or certification required for this safe natural therapy. For further reading, research, and information refer to American Health Service Magnetics, 14092 Lambs Lane, Libertyville, IL 60048.

MASSAGE THERAPY IN LIVER DISEASES

Massage therapy is perhaps the oldest and simplest alternative treatment. From past and present the ancient Chinese, Egyptian, Greek, Roman, and today's practitioners use massage to heal and relieve pain. The principle of this therapy is profound and it's accepted as a natural treatment for people of all ages.

In recent years massage therapy has shown to improve patient's morale; relieve stress; improve muscle efficiency, movement, and circulation; and promote good health and hastened a speedy recovery. Massage therapy is easy to learn. It's not limited to specific people. It is a therapy that everyone can acquire; no special equipment is required. There is no risk of dangerous side effects. It is as pleasant to give as it is to receive. The pressure used in massage, whether heavy or light, skillful or unskillful, if done correctly help the body in healing. In the case of liver disorders: You need to work on the abdomen using broad circling the belly, spiraling round the belly and long stroke, using breathing. Stretching and draining the leg is also beneficial.

Nobody knows your body as well as you do. You can use self-massage anywhere, at work or at home, whenever you are feel tense or tired, stiff or aching. For more information, contact Massage Magazine, 1315 West Mallon Avenue, Spokane, WA 99201.

AEROBIC EXERCISERS IN LIVER DISEASES

There is no doubt that regular aerobic exercise can help prevent disease. Some studies suggest that activity, even at low levels, plays as strong a role in preventing certain types of diseases such as cancer, heart disease, colon cancer, breast cancer, and stomach disorders.

One study done by researchers at a prestige university found that women who had been active in sports while in college (those who burned 2,500 or more calories a week engaging in sports) had less risk of developing breast cancer; men had low colon cancer incidence than inactive man or women who did less physical activity. Researchers aren't yet sure how exercise cuts your risk of developing disease. One theory is that exercise helps keep you lean and at your ideal body weight. Being overweight is known to increase the risk for endometrial and gall bladder cancer, breast cancer, and colon cancer.

Constipation has been linked to colon cancer, and there is evidence that inactive people are more likely to be constipated, which may increase risk of cancer. According to New York gastroenterologist Myron D. Goldberg, M.D., author of *The Inside Tract: The Complete Guide to Digestive Disorders,* "Any exercise that strengthens the abdominal muscle make it easier to pass a stool. Sweating draws from your body and may contribute to constipation. It's advisable to drink plenty of fluids if you are working up a sweat, or exercising in hot, humid weather. Also, the body's immune system affects by exercise and can help reduce the bad effects of stress-related hormone. Such hormones may be related to depressed immune functions, researchers say.

Researchers don't know yet if exercise does, in fact, help people with disease to live longer. But they do know exercise can make a big difference in how person feels. One thing for sure exercise can help prevent heart disease, build strong bones, help with your sex life, arthritis pain, prevent back pain, preserve your memory, improve the breathing problems of asthma, and prevent certain types of cancer. A study from the National Health and Nutrition Examination Survey (NHANES) compared physical activity with rates of cancer in a large number of men and women. It found that men who considered themselves inactive had nearly twice the risk of developing cancer as active men. An inactive woman had an approximately 50 percent higher risk than active women.

I suggest an aerobic exercise regime of walking, swimming, biking, or running at moderated pace for everybody. Always warm up first.

Breathe slowly and deeply, and avoid holding your breath. All you need is dedication, perseverance, determination, and practice.

Yoga Therapy in Liver Diseases

Yoga is called the mother of many forms of exercise. Does it help in liver disorders? This 5,000-year-old discipline sees the body as physical manifestation of the mind and spirit, which are interrelated as one unit. In another words, in yoga to heal the body is also to heal the mind and spirit.

Yoga masters over the centuries have contended that a yoga program can cure just about any health problem from asthma, diabetes, heart disease, arthritis, back pain, and mental disorders such as nervousness and depression, to name just a few. Today, yoga plays a major role in our lives and is practiced throughout the world.

Some studies show that yoga can change temporary the way the body functions. There is no studies show that liver diseases patient help from yoga. But, some studies show that regular yoga practices Increases strength, coordination, and stamina. If you have liver diseases practicing yoga may found very beneficial.

The safest way to practice yoga therapy is to follow a program, and there are many schools of yoga, journals, and organizations you may contact for further assistance, including the following: Samata Yoga and Health Institute, 4150 Tivoli Avenue, Los Angeles, CA 90066; Yoga Journal, 2054 University Avenue, Berkeley, CA 94704; or the International Association of Yoga Therapists, 109 Hillside Avenue, Mill Valley, CA 94941.

Nutrition in Liver Diseases

Nutrition and liver are interrelated in many ways. Everything we eat, breathe, and absorb is detoxified by the liver. This is why we call liver in natural medicine the center for detoxification. The body is the internal chemical power plant.

We know that 80 to 90 percent of the blood that leaves the stomach and intestines carries nutrients to the liver, which are then converted into substances the body can use. It processes carbohydrates, proteins, fats, and minerals to be used in maintaining normal body functions.

Can poor nutrition cause liver disease? We don't know, but with the exception of alcoholic liver disease and liver disease found among starving populations. Some researcher found good nutrition, a balanced diet with adequate calories, proteins, fats, and carbohydrates can help a damaged liver to regenerate new liver cells. In fact, in some liver disease, such as common viral hepatitis, cirrhosis, obstruction of the bile ducts, and exposure to certain drugs or toxic substances, nutrition becomes an essential form of treatment.

Adults with cirrhosis require a balanced diet rich in protein, with 2,000 to 3,000 calories daily to allow the liver cells to regenerate. Too much protein will result an increased amount in ammonia in the blood; too little protein can reduce healing of liver. A careful monitoring of protein is important by the license healthcare practitioner.

There are many others nutritional problems caused by cirrhosis when scarring of cirrhosis interferes with the flow of blood from the stomach and intestines to the liver, a condition called portal hypertension, which means that there is back pressure in the veins entering the liver. If shunting occurs to correct the problem. High levels of amino acids, ammonia and possible toxins if those compounds reach the brain, liver may caused mental impairment (confusion and loss of memory), a condition called hepatic encephalopathy. Restricting the amount of protein, sodium (salt) and food like: shellfish, canned soup and vegetables, cold cuts, dairy products and condiments like mayonnaise and ketchup, vitamin A in excess in the diet may be beneficial for the liver.

Then is other disease change in diet can help Cholestasis back up bile in the liver). Stcatouliea (Fat is not absorbed but in large amount in the fees Wilson disease (large amount of copper may build-up in the body. Homochromatosis (large amount of iron are transported from the intestines and accumulate in the liver).

Fat can be accumulated in the liver through chemicals or drugs. Nutritional causes of a fatty liver include starvation, protein malnutrition, and intestinal bypass operation for obesity, as well as certain chemical, drug compounds, and endocrine disorders. Treatment calls for addressing the related causes. To avoid a fatty liver, limit intake of alcohol and watch the diet, obesity, and weight reduction.

A low fat diet with high intake of protein (about 1 to 1.5 grams protein per kg body weight) and sufficient calories to maintain weight is recommended. Some researchers state that multivitamin and antioxidants are beneficial, but it is strongly advised not to take megavitamin without consulting a licensed healthcare practitioner.

Fiber in Liver Diseases

Fiber is important for many reasons: for the health of the digestive system, lowering the cholesterol, aiding food and waste to move through the digestive system, helping decrease the rate of blood rise after meal, and controlling the appetite by working to feel you longer.

Foods that have fiber are good sources for essential nutrients. The Food and Nutrition Boards define fiber as: dietary fiber and functional fiber with classifications of soluble (dissolve in water) and insoluble (do not dissolve in water).

Soluble fiber: oat bran, oat meal, beans, peas, rice bran, barley, citrus fruits, strawberries, and apple pulp.

Insoluble fiber: wheat breads, wheat cereals, wheat bran, rye, rice, barley, cabbage, beats, carrots, Brussels sprouts, turnips, cauliflower, and apple skin.

Many health experts are advising people of all ages to consume more dietary fiber. Much research suggests that fiber may help repair damaged liver by regenerating new cells and preventing cancer, diabetes, heart diseases, and obesity.

COMMON VITAMIN/HERBAL MISTAKES

Millions of people all over the world now take vitamin and supplements. That's a good thing. But it is very important to know if you are taking them correctly. The FDA does not require expiration dates on supplements. I recommend that if there is no expiration date, you should not buy the product. Some nutrients maintain their potency for years, others do not. Some products are so old, they are useless. Some investigators found that some brands of vitamin contained zero active ingredients when tested by independent laboratories.

Some nutritional supplements block the effect of others and certain supplements should never be taken together or taken with medicines, because they produce unsafe interactions. Some brands are just plain rip-offs as there is no quality and potency.

In the United States there are no laws governing the quality or potency of supplements. The single most important factor to look for when buying any herb for common illness is to know which herbs is very important for that illness.

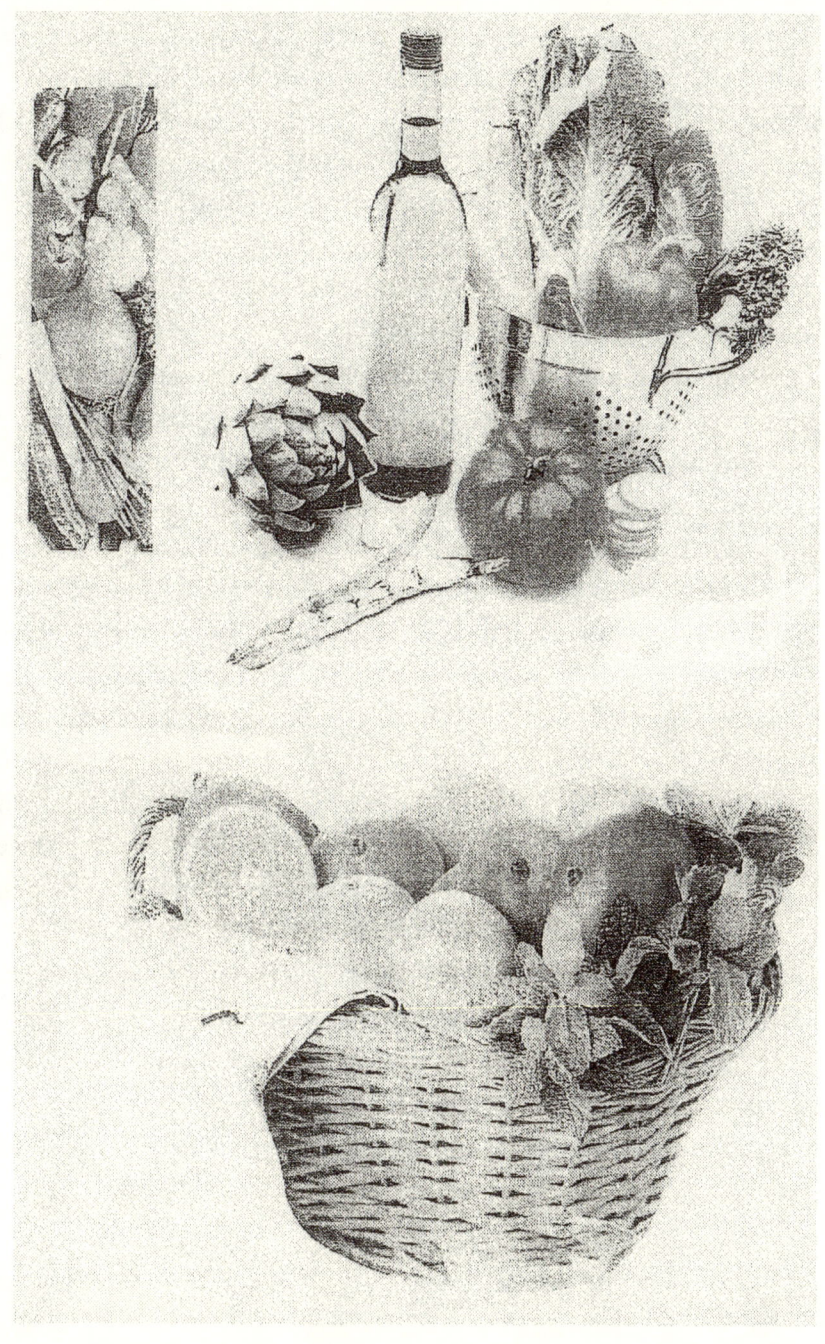

Patient Education in Liver Disorders

In several studies, liver diseases mainly hepatitis C has received broad media attention in recent years because human hepatitis C is considered curable when successfully treated. A number of studies suggest that hepatitis C virus (HCV) is now the leading cause of death in the young generation from 18 to 50 years old and the number is increasing not only in the United States but worldwide.

The best thing to do for preventing hepatitis is to participate in treatment and education programs. We see now there's hepatitis treatment education programs workshop throughout the United States. Every home should know what hepatitis is, the natural history of the disease, how it is transmitted, and conventional and alternative treatments, as well support groups.

It's good to have backup effective immune-enhancing nutrients that can triple your natural killer cells (NK) activity. Killer cells are the immune system's first line of defense. They like warriors in battle; they effectively destroy all offensive organs. There are many immune-enhancing nutrients available on the market. See your healthcare practitioner.

It is important to know that hepatitis C (HCV) and hepatitis B (HBV) may be absent of perceived symptoms until the late stage of the disease. Some individuals experience a reduction in quality of life. Therefore, everyone at risk should be tested for hepatitis B and hepatitis C, particularly if there is history injection of drug use or sex with someone who may have used intravenous drugs.

The standard of care for hepatitis C in conventional medicine is the treatment of interferon-based therapy and the most effective therapy is the combination therapy of pegylated interferon plus ribavin. Pegylated interferon is once weekly subcutaneous injection. Ribavirin pills are taken twice daily.

There are several drugs available for treatment of hepatitis C, including lamivudine (3TC), adefovir and Interferon. Although it's not approved by the FDA for the treatment of hepatitis C, Texofavir has been shown in several studies to have similar efficacy as adefovir against hepatitis C. Entecavir has been shown to be potent and effective against hepatitis C and is in the final stages of development. Studies are in progress, and the drug is expected to soon become available for the treatment hepatitis C. Treatment therapy for hepatitis C can be difficult to tolerate. Side effects such as anemia, fatigue, irritability, depression, and loss of appetite can occur.

If you have hepatitis C he can accelerate both hepatitis B and hepatitis C disease progression. Hepatitis C can be transmitted sexually but the risk is low. However, when the sex partners have a sexually transmitted diseases (STD), herpes, or open sores or engage in risky sexual behaviors such as fisting and anal sex, multiple sex partners, sex during menstruation, men who have sex with men more increased risk for transmission, they should consult with a medical doctor who specializes in treating hepatitis.

MAKING TREATMENT DECISIONS IN LIVER DISEASES

Because liver disease is the seventh leading cause of death in the United States, we need to take it seriously. The liver is one of the few organs that has the ability to repair itself and replace damaged tissue. Research in Europe, Asia, and the United States has indicated that there are many natural remedies, supplements, and diets that can stimulate regeneration of the liver cells. It is logical to think that all of us can benefit from some forms of herbal liver tonics for liver support in prevention of free radical damage and development of disease.

The Liver Disease Book of Natural Medicine focuses on hepatitis. My mission is to provide the best prevention and healing opportunities through qualities nutritional products and education materials. A record-breaking number of studies were published in the year 2000 on the ability of many herbs and nutritional products to prevent liver diseases.

For several years, researchers in Japan have been investigating the potential of ascorbic acid to enhance the ability of keeping liver enzyme to work. In Japan, glycyrrhiza glabra (licorice root) has been used in the treatment of hepatitis B. Licorice has the ability to decrease serum liver enzymes, aspartate aminotransferase (AST), and alanine aminotransferase (ALT). In a three-year study of prevention of hepatitis B in a population of 20,847 persons in Jiangsu Province, China, with supplementation of sodium selenite, the researchers concluded that the incidence of virus hepatitis infections was lower than those with no selenium.

Another report indicates the benefit of zinc and selenium of those with hepatitis. In Europe, the herb *silybuin marianum* (milk thistle) has been used as a supportive agent in the treatment of inflammatory liver diseases (hepatitis and cirrhosis).

We are fortunate today to have access to natural liver-protection remedies that are safe, effective, and without significant side effects. Lifestyle choices and personal habits will strongly impact immediate and long-term wellness. Therefore, self-awareness plays a critical role in the control of liver diseases mainly hepatitis.

All natural remedies mentioned in this book can be obtained from health food stores. No potentially harmful treatments are offered. Utilizing the healing benefits of foods and herbs can help improve our well-being. I hope The *Liver Disease Book of Natural Medicine* will be useful as well as educational.

Adams, Ruth, and Frank Murray. Complete Home Guide to Vitamins. New York: Larchmont, 1978

Adams, Rex. Mirade Medicine Foods. New York: Parker, 1977

Aikman, Lonelle. Nature's Healing Arts: From Folk Medicine to Modern Drugs. Washington, D.C.: The National Geographic Society, 1977

Ali, M., et al. Dissociation between hepatosplenic and narrow iron in liver cirrhosis. Arch. Pathol. Lab. Med., 106: 200–204, 1982

Bauer, Cathryn. Acupressure for Everybody. New York: William Morrow, 1979

Bakule, Paula Driefus, ed. Rodale's Book of Practical Formulas. Emmaus, PA: Rodale, 1991

Balch, James F., and Phyllis A. Bach. Prescriptions for Nutritional Healing. NewYork: Avery, 1990

Bell, H., and N. Raknerud, et al. Inapproppriately low levels of gonadotrophins in amenorrheac women with alcoholic and non-alcoholic cirrhosis. Eur. Endocrinol. 1995, Apr., 132 (4): 444–449

Berger, S. M. Dr. Berger's Power Diet. New York: New American Library, 1985

Bieler, Henry G., M.D. Food Is Your Best Medicine. New York: Ballantine Books, 1965

Beinfield, Harriet, and Efrem Korngold. Between Heaven and Earth: A Guide to Chinese Medicine. New York: Ballantine Books, 1991

Boss-Hamburger, Hilde. The Creative Power of Colour. London: The Michael Press, 1973

Carper Jean. The Food Pharmacy. New York: Bantam Books, 1988.

Clarke, J. H. Dictionary of Materia Medica. Essex, England: Health Sciences Press, 1987

Cameron, Myra. Life Encyclopedia of Natural Remedies. Parker Publishing copy, 1993

Carrol, David. The Complete Book of Natural Medicines. New York: Summit Books, 1980

Cumston, Charles Greene. An Introduction to the History of Medicine. New York: Dorset Press, 1987

Coulter, Hams L. Divided Legacy. Berkeley, California: Homeopathic Educational Services, 1982

Cohen, M. R. New York: The Berkley Publishing Group, 1996

Concorang, Wong B. Role of glutathlone in prevention of acetaminophen-induced hepatotoxicity by N-acetyl-D-cysteine in mice. J. Pharmacology Exp. Ther. 1986; 238:54–56

Costello, C. H., and E. V. Lynn 1950. Journal of the American Pharmaceutical Association 39:177

Cichoke A. The effect of systemic enzyme therapy on cancer cells and the immune system. Thousand letter for doctors and patients Nov. 1995:30–32 (review)

Diploc, A. Antioxidant nutrients and disease prevention: An overview. Am. J. Clin. Nutr. 53:189s;1991

Duke, J. A., Ph.D. The Green Pharmacy. New York: St. Martin's Press, 1997

De Waal, M. Medicinal Herbs in the Bible. York Beach, Maine: Samuel Weiser, 1984

De Simone C, Vesley R. Bianchi S. B., et al. The role of probiotics in modulation of the immune system in man and in animals. International Journal Immunotherapy 1993; 9:23–28

Faasati P., and M. Fassati, et al. Treatment of stabilized liver cirrhosis by dehydroepiandrostterone. Agressologia 14 (4), 1973; 259–268

Fehe J. Larry I et al. Free radicals in tissue damage in liver diseases and therapeutic approach. Tokai J. Exp. Clin. Med. 1986; 11: 121–134

Galean, Dorothy. Grandma's Remedies. Springdale, Utah: Publishing, 1987

Griffith, H. Winter. The Complete Guide to Vitamins, Minerals, Supplements, and Herbs. Tucson: Fisher Books, 1988

Griggs, Barbara. Green Pharmacy. New York: Viking, 1982. Reprinted. Rochester, VT.: Healings Arts Press, 1991

Grossman, Richard. The Other Medicines. Garden City, New York: Doubleday and Company, 1985

Hagman B, W. Ryd, and H. Skomedal. Arabinogalactan blockade of experimental metastases to liver by murine hepatoma. Invasion Metastasis. 1991; 1 1:348–355

Hausman, Patricia, and Judith Benn Hurley. The Healing Foods. Emmaus, PA: Rodale Press, 1989

Hendler, Shendler Saul, M.D., Ph.D. The Doctor's Vitamin and Mineral Encyclopedia. New York: Simon and Schuster, 1990

Hobbs, C. Medicinal Mushrooms. Santa Cruz, CA: Botanica Press, 1995

Hill, Howard E. Introduction to Lecithin. New York: Pyramid, 1972

Hunt, Roland T. The Eight Keys to Colour. London: L. N. Fowler and Co, Ltd., 1965

Kaptchuk, Ted. The Web that Has No Weaver. New York: Congdon and Weed, 1983

Kent, J. T. Lectures on Homeopathic Materia Medica. New Delhi: Blain Publishers, 1982

Keys, John D., Chinese Herbs Tokyo, Japan: Charles E. Tuttle Company, 1993

Lust, John. The Herb Book. New York: Bantam Books, 1974

Mabey, Richard. The New Age Herbalist. New York: MacMillan Co., 1988

Mills, Simon Y., ed. The Dictionary of Modern Herbalism. A Comprehensive Guide to Practical Herbal Therapy. Rochester, Vermont: Healing Press, 1988

Oetel, G. J. Effect of moderate exercise on bowel habit. Gut 1991;32: 941–944

Prevention Magazine staff. Lifespan Plus. Emmaus, PA: Rodale, 1990

Prevention Magazine staff. The Complete Book of Vitamins.
  Emmaus, PA: Rodale, 1977, 1984

Rice-Evans, C. Free Radicals, Cell Damage, and Disease. London:
  Richelieu Press, 1986

Rudolf, F. W., M.D. Herbal Medicine. The Bath Press, 1982

Reid, Daniel P. Chinese Herbal Medicine. Boston: Shambhale, 1987

Soule, Deb. The Roots of Healing. New York: Citadel Press, 1995

Simons, Anne, M.D., Bobbie Hasselbring, and Michael Castleman.
  Before you call the doctor

Strehlow, Wighard, and Gottfried Hertzka. Hidegard of Bengen's
  Medicine. Santa Fe, New Mexico: Bear and Co., 1988

Stone, Irwin. The Healing Factor: Vitamin C Against Disease. New
  York: Pitman, 1971

Sumioka, I., T. Matsura, and K. Yamada. Therapeutic Effect of S-
  Allylmercaptocysteine on acetaminophen-induced liver injury
  in mice. Eur. J. Pharmacology 2001. Dec 21: 433 (2–3): 177–
  185

Tang, Stephen, and Martin Palmer. Chinese Herbal Prescriptions.
  London: Rider and Company, 1987

Tyler, M. L. Pointers to the Common Remedies. New Delhi: Blain
  Publishers, 1988

Tkac, Debora, ed. The Doctors Book of Home Remedies. Emmaus,
  PA: Rodale, 1990

Uri, Lloyd. King's American Dispensatory, 18th edition, 1898.
  Portland, Oregon: Electric Medical Publications, 1983

Veith, Ilza, trans. The Yellow Emperor's Classic of Internal Medicine.
  Berkeley: University of California Press, 1966

Weil, Andrew, M.D. Spontaneous Healing. New York: Alfred A.
  Knopf, 1995

Weil, Andrew, M.D. Natural Health, Natural Medicine. Boston:
  Houghton-Mifflin, 1996

Williams, Roger. Nutrition Against Disease. New York: Pitman, 1971

William, Terry. Textbook of Modern Herbology. Calgary, Alberta:
  Progressive Publishing, 1988

Yeung, Him-Che. Handbook of Chinese Herbs and Formulas. Los Angeles: Institute of Chinese Medicine, 1985

U.S DEPARTMENT OF HEALTH & HUMAN SERVICES
Center for Disease Control and Prevention

WHAT YOU NEED TO KNOW ABOUT
VIRAL HEPATITIS RISK

Top 11 Most Frequently Asked Questions About Viral Hepatitis

Reprint from : http ;//www.cdc.gov/ncidod/diseases/hepatitis/commom-faqs.htm
Division of Viral Hepatitis – center for Disease Control and Prevention National
Center for Infections Diseases

<u>What is viral hepatitis?</u>

<u>What are the symptoms of viral hepatitis?</u>

<u>How are hepatitis A, B, and C viruses spread?</u>

Hepatitis A Virus (HAV)

Hepatitis B Virus (HBV)

Hepatitis C Virus (HCV)

<u>Can I donate blood if I have had any type of viral hepatitis?</u>

<u>How long can HAV, HBV and HCV survive outside the body?</u>

Hepatitis A Virus (HAV)

Hepatitis Virus B (HBV)

Hepatitis C (HCV)

<u>For how long is hepatitis B vaccine effective?</u>

<u>Are booster of hepatitis B vaccine needed?</u>

<u>What does the term " hepatitis B carrier " mean?</u>

<u>If my hepatitis B vaccination series is interrupted, do I have to start over?</u>

<u>What is the treatment for chronic hepatitis B?</u>

<u>What is the treatment for chronic hepatitis C?</u>

WHAT IS VIRAL HEPATITIS?

Hepatitis means inflammation of the liver. Viral hepatitis is inflammation of the liver caused by a virus. There are five identified types of viral hepatitis and each one is caused by a different virus. In the United States, hepatitis A, hepatitis B and hepatitis C are the most common types.

Hepatitis A is caused by hepatitis A virus (HAV), hepatitis B virus (HBV), and hepatitis C is caused by hepatitis C virus (HCV).

tiredness

loss of appetite

nausea

abdominal discomfort

dark urine

clay-colored bowel movements

yellowing of the skin and eyes (jaundice)

HOW ARE HEPATITIS A, B, AND C VIRUSES SPREAD ?

HEPATITIS A VIRUS (HAV)

Hepatitis A virus is spread from person to person by putting something in the mouth that has been contaminated with the stool of a person with hepatitis A. This type of transmission is called "fecal-oral." Most infections result from contact with a household member or sex partner who is infected with HAV. Casual contact, as in the usual office, factory, or school setting, does not spread the virus.

HEPATITIS B VIRUS (HBV)

HBV is spread when blood or body fluids from an infected person enters the body of a person who is not infected. For example, HBV is spread through having sex with an infected person without using a condom (the efficacy of latex condoms in preventing infection with HBV is unknown, but their proper use might reduce transmission), by sharing drugs, needles, or "works" when "shooting" drugs, through needlesticks or sharps exposures on the job, or from an infected mother to her baby during birth.

HEPATITIS C VIRUS (HCV)

HCV is spread when blood or body fluids from an infected person enters the body of a person who is not infected. This could happen through sharing needles or"works" when "shooting" drugs, through needlesticks or sharps exposures on the job, or from an infected mother to her baby during birth.

CAN I DONATE BLOOD IF I HAVE HAD ANY TYPE OF VIRAL HEPATITIS?

If you had any type of viral hepatitis since age 11, you are not eligible to donate blood. In addition, if you ever tested positive for hepatitis B or hepatitis C, at any age, you are not eligible to donate, even if you were never sick or jaundiced from the infection.

HOW LONG CAN HAV, HBV AND HCV SURVIVE OUTSIDE THE BODY?

HAV

HAV can live outside the body for months, depending on the environmental conditions.

HBV

HBV can survive outside the body at least 7 days and still be capable of transmitting infection

HCV

Recent studies have shown that HCV can survive outside the body and still transmit infection for 16 hours, but not longer than 4 days.

FOR HOW LONG IS HEPATITIS B VACCINE EFFECTIVE?

Long – term studies of healthy adults and children indicate that hepatitis B vaccine protects against chronic HBV infection for at least 15 years, even though antibody levels might decline below detectable levels.

ARE BOOSTER OF HEPATITIS B VACCINE NEEDED?

No, booster doses of hepatitis B vaccine are not recommended routinely.

Data show that vaccine-induced hepatitis B surface antibody (anti-HBS) levels might decline over time; however, immune memory (anamnestic anti-HBs response) remains intact indefinitely following immunization. People with declining antibody levels are still protected against clinical illness and chronic disease.

WHAT DOES THE TERM " HEPATITIS B CARRIER" MEAN?

"Hepatitis B carrier" is a term that is sometimes used to indicate people who have chronic (long term) infection with HBV, Two percent to 6% of persons over 5 years of age; 30% of children 1 – 5 years of age; and up to 90% of infants develop chronic infection. Persons with chronic infection can infect others and are at increased risk of serious liver disease including cirrhosis and liver cancer. In the United States, an estimated 1.25 million people are chronically infected with HBV.

If my hepatitis B vaccination series is interrupted, do I have to start over?

No. If the vaccination series is interrupted, resume with the next dose in the series.

What is the treatment for chronic hepatitis B?

There are three drugs licensed for the treatment of persons with chronic hepatitis B: Adefovir dipivoxil, alpha interferon, and lamivudine.

What is the treatment for hepatitis C?

Combination therapy, using pegylated interferon and ribavirin, is currently the treatment of choice.